THE RE-CENTER METHOD NATURAL DIET
SALAD BOOK

Celebrate the Joy of Salad International Recipes from 7 Continents to boost your metabolism in Just 21 Days

Hareldau Argyle King

Also Available from Refinement Publishing & Media

Quotes to Habits
Remember
Hareldau Argyle King

The Re-center Method
Natural Diet
Hareldau Argyle King

The Re-center Method
Natural Diet Cookbook
Hareldau Argyle King

The Re-center Method
Natural Diet Soupbook
Hareldau Argyle King

The Re-center Method
Natural Diet Smoothies
Hareldau Argyle King

© Copyright September 2022
by Refinement Publishing & Media
Published by Refinement Publishing &Media - All rights reserved.

Web site: www.beingelevatedlifestyle.com
Email: support@beingelevatedlifestyle.com

As with all exercises and dietary programs, you should get your doctor's approval before beginning. The information here is to help you make an informed decision about your health.

This book is not intended as a substitute for any treatment that may have been prescribed by your doctor. The reader should regularly consult a doctor in matters about his/her health and particularly concerning any symptoms that may require diagnosis or medical attention.

This book is intended as a reference manual and not a medical manual. The exercises and dietary programs in the book are not intended as a substitute for any exercise routine or dietary regimen that may have been prescribed by your doctor.

Copyright © 2022 by Refinement Publishing &Media
All rights reserved.

All rights reserved. No part of the publication may be reproduced or transmitted in any form or by any means. Without the express written permission of the publisher except for the use of brief quotations in a book review.

The scanning, uploading, and distribution of this book via the internet or any other means without the permission of the publisher are illegal and punishable by law. Please by law Please purchase only authorized electronic editions and do not participate in or encourage electronic piracy of copyrighted materials. Your support of the author's rights is appreciated.

www.beingelevatedlifestyle.com
ISBN 978-1-950838-24-0 Ebook
ISBN- 978-1-9508 38-25-7 Hardcover
ISBN 978-1-950838-26-4 Paperback

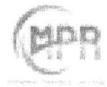

ACKNOWLEDGMENTS

Meals taste better when shared in the community, and even better when shared with stories among family, friends, and colleagues.

I am grateful for every friend, family member, and & passing acquaintance I shared a unique meal, whether the meals were a local dish or an elaborate international meal.

Whether it was served at a dinner party, upscale restaurant, a local diner, or a backyard cookout. In every city I lived, town I passed through, and country every visited I say Thank you.

Your generosity encouraged me to gather & create this collection of recipes from different states and nations.

FOREWORD

Hareldau and I have known each other for a lifetime. When she embarked on this project, I was so excited and thrilled for her.

Since our days in Atoms Athletic Club in Guyana, she has always had big dreams and aspirations and our club was supportive of her dreams.

All through our years in Washington DC and New York City, she managed to stay focused and hold on to the love for good foods, people, interesting conversations, and a life full of adventures.

This book will open your world to some interesting, appetizing, and mind-blowing recipes that will be a must-have at your social gathering, dinner tables, and just to have daily.

I don't have a favorite recipe they all are good.

I urge you as have fun with these recipes. They have been gathered and influenced by some very fascinating global citizens that she has met over the years

Enter an adventure for your pallet!

Cheers

Angilla Nicky Corlette

Gourmet educator

DEDICATION

IN HONOR OF
ANGILLA NICKY CORLETTE

In honor of my dear childhood friend, international track athlete and gourmet educator
Ms. Angilla Nicky Corlette loves for food, family & fun is infectious
You are a source of calm, comfort, and delightful cuisine.
A kind soul, kindred spirit, a caring friend.
Your relentlessness for living, simplicity to challenges and curiosity for new recipes, exotic cuisine and fine dining inspires me daily.
I applaud the years of investment you have made in studying, practicing, and teaching the science of food and its preparation.
Our Friendship is invaluable!

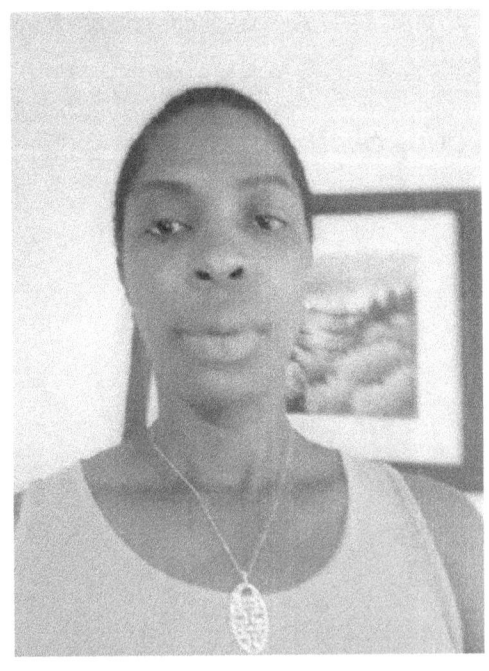

Angilla Nicky Corlette

How to Use this Book

This book is a guide to a higher quality of life, through building relationships and varying your food choices. Whether you never had an international meal or friend or whether this is your way of life, there are words of encouragement, new ideas & solutions to enhance your quality of life.

The book is divided into 5 sections. The first section is Green Salad recipes. Section II consists of Vegetable Salad recipes, Section III Pasta salads recipes and Section Iv Legumes, meat or grains-mixed salads and Section v fruit salad recipes from 7 continents.

If you notice a country under a different classification, it may be because some countries may be geographically located in one continent as well as cultural associate with another.

This is not a diet book, a weight loss book, or a meal plan. On your first attempt to prepare these dishes, your meal may or may not look like the photo of the meal in this book.

This book is designed to enhance your taste bud, exposing you to different textures and tastes of food from all the continents of the world. After you would complete this 4-part of series international recipe books you experience cuisines from 195 countries in 7 continents.

I invite you to get started today. Don't Procrastinate!!

Table of Content

Introduction..1

Section: 1 Green Salad..5

Latin America & the Caribbean..6

Belize: Belizean Salad...7
Nicaragua: Nicaraguan Green Salad..8
Argentina: Argentinean Green Salad..10
Bolivia: Bolivian Carrot and Lettuce Salad..11
Brazil: Brazilian Salad..12
Cuba: Cuban Cabbage and Cilantro Salad..13
Dominican Republic: Beetroot Salad...14
Haiti: Haitian Salad...15
Guadeloupe: Green Salad..16
Martinique : Parisian Salad..17

Asia

Indonesia: Indonesian Salad..18
Myanmar: Burmese Cabbage Salad...19
Vietnam: Vietnamese Salad...20
China: Chinese Salad..21

Australia & Oceania

Australia: Australian Salad..22
Kiribati: Kiribati Salad...23
Micronesia: Micronesian Salad...24
Burkina Faso: Burkina Faso Salad...25

Africa

Burundi: Burundian Salad...26
Egypt: Egyptian Salad..27
Comoros: Comorian Salad..28
Côte d'Ivoire: Cote d' Ivoire Salad....................................29

North America

Newfoundland, Canada: Newfoundland Potato Salad.........30
Los Cabos, Mexico: Special Salad....................................31
Acapulco, Mexico: Acapulco Salad..................................32
Veracruz, Mexico: Veracruz Salad...................................33
Boston, Massachusetts: Boston Salad.............................34
St Louis, Missouri: Vegetable Salad................................35

Europe

Italy: Italian Salad..36
Andorra: Chicory Salad..37
Liechtenstein: Liechtenstein Salad.................................38
San Marino: San Marina Salad.......................................39
Holy See: Holy See Salad...40

Section: 11 Vegetable Salads...41

Latin America & The Caribbean

Panama: Panama Salad..42
Costa Rica: Costa Rican Salad.......................................43
Chile: Chilean Salad...44
Colombia: Columbian Salad...45
Ecuador: Ecuadorian Salad..46
Puerto Rico: Puerto Rico Salad......................................47
Saint-Barthélemy: Saint-Barthélemy Salad....................48
Saint-Martin: Saint Martin Salad....................................49
Jamaica: Jamaican Salad...50
Trinidad & Tobago: Trinidadian Potato Salad.................51

Asia

Tajikistan: Tajikistan Salad 'Qurtob'......82
Uzbekistan: Lagman Uzbek Noodle Salad......83
Afghanistan: Afghan Pasta Salad......84
Bangladesh: Bengali Pasta Salad......85
Bhutan: Britain Pasta Salad......86

Australia & Oceania

Fiji: Fiji Pasta Salad......87
Marshall Islands: Special salad......88

Africa

Mali: Curry Noodle Salad......89
Mauritius: Mauritius salad......90
Namibia: Namibian Salad......91
Niger: Niger pasta salad......92
Chad: Chad salad......93

North America

Saskatchewan, Canada: Pasta Salad......94
Guadalajara, Mexico: Elbow Pasta Salad......95
Huatulco, Mexico: Pasta Salad......96
Las Vegas Nevada: Vegetable Pasta Salad......97
Charleston, West Virginia: Pasta Salad......98

Europe

Ukraine: Ukrainian pasta salad......99
Romania: Romanian salad......100
Netherlands: Netherland salad......101
Austria: Austrian Salad......102
Serbia: Serbia salad......103

Section iv: Legumes, Meat or Grains-Mixed Salads......104

Guatemala: Special Cucumber, bean, watermelon, and feta salad......105

Peru: Chickpeas, spinach, and tomato salad...106
Suriname: Special Fava bean salad..107
Saint Lucia: Lentil salad with olives and tuna...108
Aruba: Shrimp and chickpea salad..109
United States Virgin Islands: American pasta and bean salad.......................110
Antigua and Barbuda: Cucumber, beans and feta cheese salad....................111
Dominica: Dominican salad..112

Asia

The Maldives: Maldeev tuna salad mashuni..113
Nepal: Nepali salad..114
Sri Lanka: Sri Lankan Salad...115
Iran: Iran legume salad..116
Jordan: Jordanian Salad..117

Australia & Oceania

Palau: Legume salad..118
Papua New Guinea: Special lettuce and bean sprouts salad.........................119
Samoa: Decorated salad..120

Africa

Senegal: Senegalese Salad..121
Seychelles: Seychelles salad..122
Somalia: Somalian salad...123
Burundi: Mixed beans and corn salad...124
Tunisia: Tunisian salad...125

North America

British Columbia, Canada: British Columbia salad.......................................126
Mexico City, Mexico: Mexico bean salad..127
San Cristobel de las Casas, Mexico: San Cristobel de las Casas, Mexico Sal.128
Detroit Michigan: Detroit Special corn salad...129
Phoenix, Arizona: Phoenix, Arizona salad..130

Europe

Slovenia: Slovenian Salad 131
Latvia: Latvian Salad 132
Estonia: Salad "Chick-chick" 133
Malta: Mediterranean Salad 134

Section v: Fruit Salads 135

Latin America & The Caribbean

Honduras: Waldorf salad 136
Uruguay: Uruguay Salad 137
Venezuela: Venezuela Salad 138
Cayman Islands: Cayman Islands Salad 139
Saint Kitts And Nevis: Chicken and mixed fruit salad 140
Turks and Caicos Islands: Island Salad 141
Saint Martin: Tropical Fruit Salad 142
British Virgin Islands: BVI Salad 143
Anguilla: Anguilla Salad 144

Asia

Syria: Syrian Salad 145
Yemen: Yemen Salad 146
South Korea: South Korea Salad 147
Brunei: Brunei Salad 148

Australia & Oceania

Solomon Islands: Solomon Islands Salad 149
Tonga: Tonga Salad 150
Vanuatu: Vanuatu Salad 151

Africa

South Sudan: South Sudan Salad 152
Sudan: Canned fruit salad 153
Cape Verde: Cape Verde Salad 154
Libya: Libya Salad 155

North America

Nunavut Canada: Chicken and mixed fruit salad...156
Puebla, Mexico: Cinnamon apple salad...157
Playa del Carmen, Mexico: Special avocado salad..158
Philadelphia, PA: Cream cheese fruit salad...159

Europe

France: French fruit salad...160
Belarus: Belarus Fresh Strawberries...161
Kosovo: Kosovo Salad..162
Iceland: Fresh Fruit Salad...163
Bulgaria: Bulgaria Papayas Salad..164
Next Step...165

INTRODUCTION

Dear Friend,

Celebrating the joy of healthy eating of global cuisine is essential for a sustainable lifestyle.

When was the last time you had a new food experience? Cooked a new healthy meal, dined at different exotic international restaurants, or shopped at a specialty supermarket?

Embracing different textures, types, and touches of food adds to living a full, fit, and fun lifestyle.

It is often said that books you read or don't read reflect your mindset, your bank, and your credit card statement since reflecting your priorities and what you value. Glancing into your shopping basket at the grocery store or farmer's market reflects your waistline, your taste bud, and your food tendencies.

As a fitness professional, nutrition specialist, and food & culture enthusiast, I am constantly observing other people's food habits in grocery stores and restaurants while managing my own. I find myself curiously observing other people's shopping habits in the checkout aisle, much the way friends and family come over to examine what's on my plate and in glass at a cocktail or dinner party. A wiser statement a friend said to me about food choices is "every time I do grocery shopping, I purchase at least one item I have never tried before" This statement inspires me every day.

A glance into your shopping cart will tell me where you spend most of your time shopping and the quality of the food you are buying, whether it is in between the aisle getting lots of cans, frozen meals, and bagged snacks or on the perimeter of the store getting fresh fruits & vegetables, lean cuts of meats or you explored the international aisle add some variety to your healthy meals.

In college is where my love language of international cuisines & curiosities started. I went to school with students from many nations while sticking to a healthy southern meal plan of cafeteria food for track athletes and surviving the tortuous bayou heat. I was starting to desire geera, masala, curry, jerk, and other tantalizing flavors.

I intentionally started seeking out international students making new friends and embracing new cultures. It was my low-budget way of gathering recipes, tasting new cuisines, and sharing stories about the uniqueness of culture from people from around the world. I quickly discovered almost every culture has a unique way of preparing two things: bread and rice & peas.

I was intentional about making new friends, I think I met and had a friend from almost every nation that was represented on the LSU campus. I can still remember the taste, the stories shared, and many friends as we connected over meals. We didn't have many resources, and we didn't have much time, yet we found a way to tear down walls of isolation and build bridges with each other through food and stories about family and traditions.

This book is a continuation of the food experiences that have profoundly changed and shaped my lifestyle. This collection of recipes gathered is in a 4-part series. Part 1 – Cookbook, part 2- A

Soup book, part 3- Salad book, and Part 4 Smoothie book a total of 195 countries that will be released over 12 months period. It is a gift I have been given in college I now give to you.

Have you ever wondered how unpleasant life would be without good food? Food is an essential requirement for growth and tissue repair. It's equally important that you make nutritious food choices.

It has been proposed that breakfast is the most important food for the day. A healthy choice is another factor. Better breakfast options include a mix of protein, healthy fat, and fiber with little or no added sugar. The food eaten upon waking is used to refuel the body after a prolonged night of fasting and sets the pace for the rest of the day.

Each meal in the day is important to attain and sustain a healthy lifestyle. Research shows that people who eat breakfast have lesser consumption of calories throughout the day, are more likely to gain healthier muscle weight, and are less likely to experience morning fatigue and emotional instabilities.

Lunch is another important part of a day's meal. This is because eating in the afternoon replenishes the depleted energy reserves to enable you to regain focus through the activities of the day. It also supplies glucose to the blood for healthy brain function.

Dinner completes the daily food intake that may be inadequate during the day. Dinner must be also nutritious and lean; to help prepare the body that is going resting stage for a good night's sleep and recovery.

A lifestyle of healthy living is a celebration of healthy eating. Food is good its purpose is to fuel the body with energy to do work, work in the gym or the field, work in the office or at home.

Food is also used as a connector, whether among friends at school in the cafeteria or colleagues at lunch in the office or among families at dinner.

This cookbook consists of 154 recipes for salad.

I invite you to explore each continent and all the nations. That exploration journey starts in this cookbook, and leads to the international aisle in the supermarket, on towards your table and table bud. The ultimate hope is that this new healthy food experience would lead to purchasing a ticket to visit a nation, build connections and make new friends along the way. If for some reason you are unable to travel to another country because of time, money, safety, or the borders are chosen because of a health crisis. You still have an opportunity to experience a new food experience, a new way of eating, and a new way of living through the pages of this book. The Re-center Method Natural Diet Salad book.

Celebrating the joy of healthy eating of global cuisine is essential for a sustainable lifestyle.

Joyfully

Hareldau Argyle King

Founder of Being Elevated Lifestyle

Section 1

Green Salad

Start with a base of leafy greens
Add crunchy ingredients
Add herbs
Add cheese
Dress it up
Make a green salad for lunch or dinner

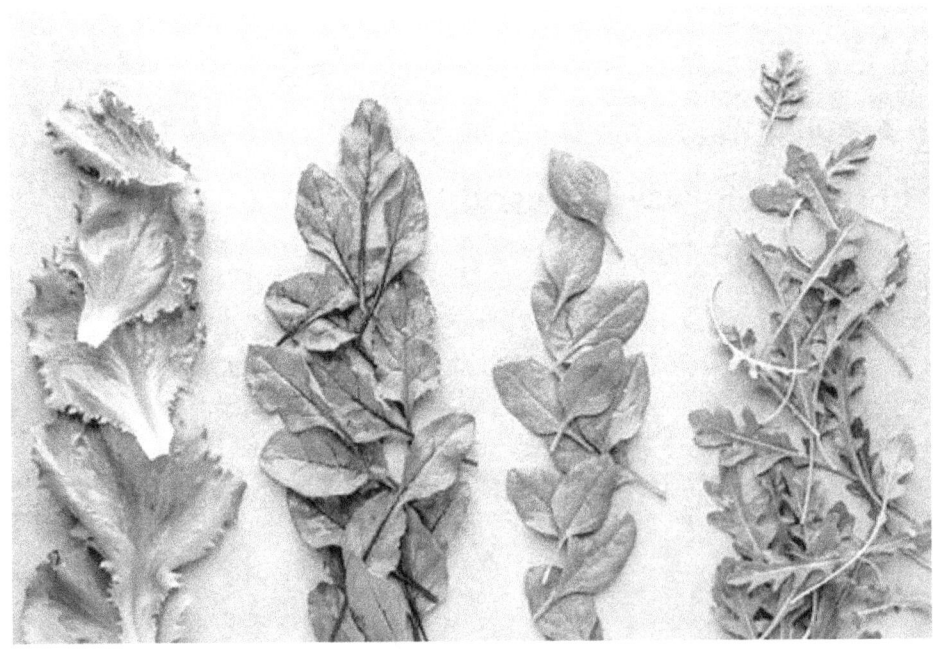

Latin America & the Caribbean

This group of countries is home to a diverse range of countries and to some of the world's most important ecosystems. The countries have a wide range of natural resources and biodiversity, many types of animals, cuisine and people each with their own culture and traditions; it is an excellent place for nature lovers.

The most widely spoken languages are English, Spanish, French and Portuguese and Dutch.

Belize: Belizean Salad

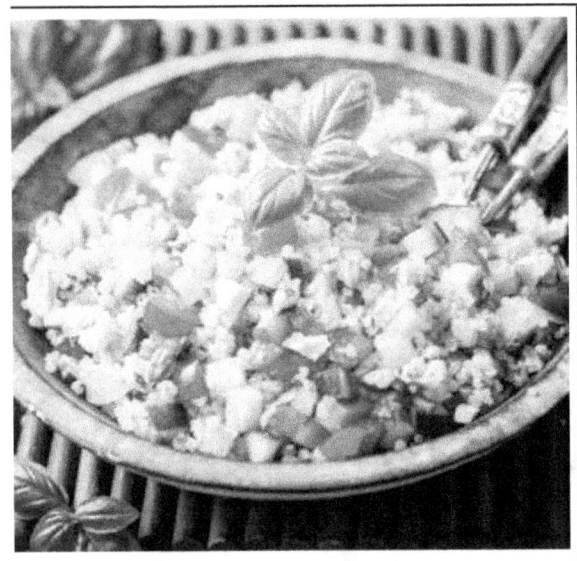

Belize

Belizean people are known for their warmth, friendliness, and sense of humor. Tourism is major source of income.

Belize is the only English-speaking country in central America with large mixture of people and traditions.

Corn, barbecued chicken, corn and tortillas are famed foods of Belize. They also serve rum with coconut water as their traditional drink

INGREDIENTS

- A 450g can of pineapple slices
- Diced cucumber 1 cup medium sized
- Parsley or cilantro a handful
- Spinach 1 cup
- Green onions 2 chopped

DIRECTIONS

1. Drain the pineapple and separate the juice in another bowl.
2. Toss all the ingredients in a salad bowl.
3. Pour 4 tab spoon of reserved pineapple can juice, salt, black pepper. Squeeze some lemon juice.
4. Mix until all well combined.
5. Chill in refrigerator for 25 minutes and enjoy!

Nicaragua: Nicaraguan Green Salad

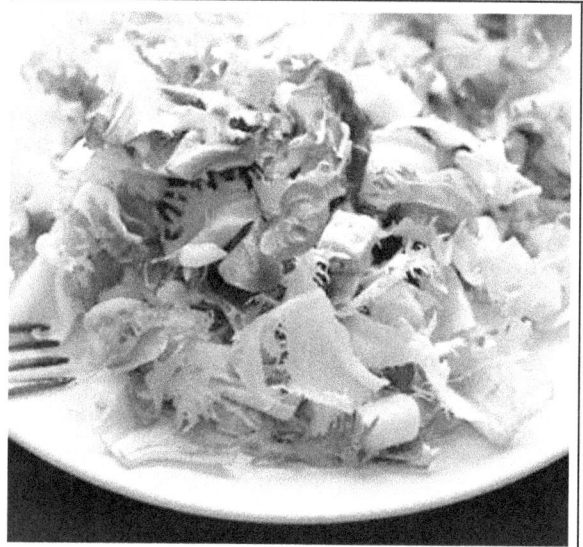

INGREDIENTS

- Savory, shreddedcabbage ½ cup
- Cooked and Peeled cassava 1//2 cup
- Chopped parsley 3 tbsp
- Chopped chives 2 tbsp
- Lime juice 2 tbsp.
- Apple 1 sliced
- Onion 1 small-sized chopped
- Salt 1/4teaspoon.
- Black pepper ¼ tsp
- Tomato 1 chopped
- Olive oil 1 tab spoon.
- Pork rinds 1 cup.
- Classic French dressing 2 tbsp
- Special coleslaw dressing 1 /4 cup and 1 tbsp.
- For serving Banana leaves
- French dressing
- Ingredients.
- Olive oil 1/2 cup
- Vinegar 2 tbsp spoon.

Nicaragua

Nicaragua is beautiful country of beaches an lakes attracting tourists from across the world. Nicaragua is the largest country of Central America, bordering Costa Rica, and Honduras.
Nicaragua's national dish is Gallo pinto-fried rice mixed with beans and spices. The regional drink is Gaubal (banana, milk, coconut water, and sugar).
It is home to Lake Nicaragua and Lake Managua.
Spanish is the official language with a mixture of Spanish and indigenous dishes and people.

DIRECTIONS

1. Mix flour, sugar, mustard, and vinegar, and cook for 10 minutes on low flame.
2. Beat egg and butter well.
3. Stir in prepared hot sauce.
4. Beat until the mixture gets thick.
5. Cool down and stir in cream.
6. Chill and then use in this recipe

Instructions.

1. Cut cassava into small cubes.
2. Add shredded cabbage, chopped apple, onion, tomato, parsley, chives, salt, and black Pepper in a bowl and mix well.
3. Mix both dressings and pour over the salad.
4. Presentation

- Salt ¼ teaspoon
- Crushed Black Pepper 1/4 teaspoon.
- Garlic clove 1/2
- Ice cube 1

Instructions.

- Shake all ingredients in an air-tight jar.
- Freeze for 15 minutes, then discard garlic.
- Coleslaw dressing.
- White vinegar 1 cup.
- Flour 1 teaspoon
- Salt 1 teaspoon
- Sugar 1 tab spoon.
- Butter 1 teaspoon
- Mustard powder 1/2 teaspoon.
- Egg 2 tbsp spoon.
- Cream 1/2 up.

1. Serve in banana leave, put some cassava and cooked pork rind, then pour prepared salad.
2. Chill and serve.

Argentina: Argentinean Green Salad

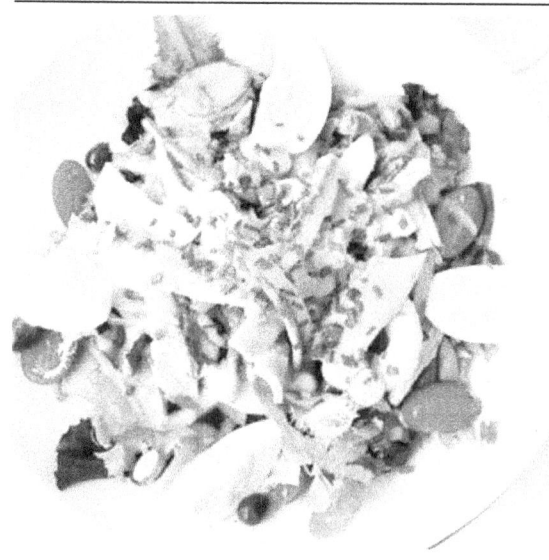

Argentina

Argentina capital is Buenos Aires with a rich cultural heritage of people, cuisine and culture.

Argentina is in the scenery southern part of South America.

There are various places to explore in Buenos Aires, from art galleries to city museums. Patagonia is an excellent place for outdoor activities such as hiking, camping, and fishing.

INGREDIENTS

- 1 head of crisp lettuce small sized.
- Tomato
- Carrot chopped 1
- Green olives 10
- Walnuts chopped 1/4 cup.
- Hard-boiled eggs 2 cut into 2 pieces.
- Parsley chopped 2 tbsp
- Chives chopped 2 tbsp
- French dressing 1/2 cup

DIRECTIONS

1. Chop lettuce leaf into bite-sized pieces.
2. Place lettuce pieces, eggs, walnuts, green olives, and carrots in a serving salad bowl.
3. Sprinkle salt and black Pepper and pour French dressing. Toss all ingredients well and serve.
4. Toss all ingredients well and serve.

Bolivia: Bolivian Carrot and Lettuce Salad

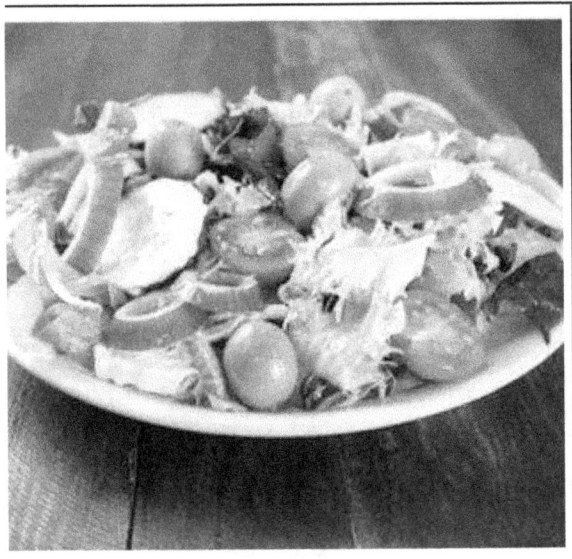

INGREDIENTS

- Lettuce 1 cup
- Tomato 1/2 cup chopped
- Carrots 2 chopped
- Onion 1 julienne cut
- Lemon juice 2 tab spoon.
- Parsley chopped 1`tab spoon
- Chives 1 tab spoon
- Olives 10
- Olive oil or salad oil ½ cup.

Bolivia

Bolivia is commonly known as a country of native people with the capital cities are Sucre and La Paz. The climate there remains relatively the same.

Bolivia's main courses and some street foods are Pique a lo macho (a combo of grilled meat with tomato and onion), Fritanga (fried pork), Salchipapa (sausages with fried potatoes).

Vitaminico, Mocochinchi, Api and Vitima with coca leaves are served as the traditional drinks.

Bolivia is a city with cheap rates for eating outside, accommodation and travelling.

DIRECTIONS

1. Mix all vegetables in a bowl.
2. Sprinkle some salt, black Pepper, parsley, and chives.
3. Blend olive oil and lemon juice until well combined.
4. Drizzle dressing onto the salad
5. Refrigerate for 15-20 minutes and serve.

Brazil: Brazilian Salad

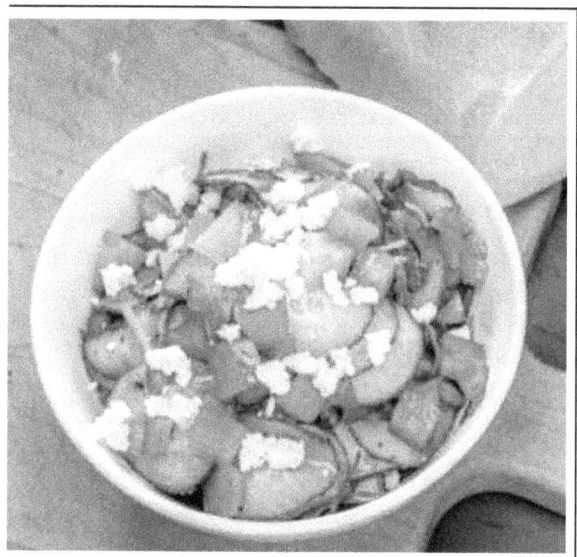

Brazil

Brazil is the largest country in South America. Brazil is a land of contrasts-Amazon Rainforest and the city of Rio de Janeiro. Popular dishes are Feijoada (meat cooked with black beans and herbs), Coxinha (croquette), Empanadas (prawn or chicken pastry pies).
The national alcohol is cachaça.
Planning a trip to Brazil check out Paraty, Rio de Janeiro, Iguazu Falls, The Pantanal, Salvador de Bahia and The Amazon Rainforest

INGREDIENTS

- Tomatoes 7 diced medium sized.
- Cucumber 3 julienne cut
- Celery 1/2 cup
- Green bell pepper 1 julienne cut.
- Spring onion 1 cup
- Lettuce 1 cup
- Parsley or chopped cilantro 2 tbs
- Dressing
- Olive oil 2 tab spoon.
- Lemon juice or apple cider vinegar 1 tab spoon
- Crushed garlic 1 teaspoon.

DIRECTIONS

1. Mix cucumbers, tomatoes, lettuce, green bell peppers, spring onions, celery, lemon juice, olive oil, cilantro, vinegar or apple cider vinegar, black Pepper, and salt in a large bowl
2. Chill in refrigerator for 1/2 hour.

Cuba: Cuban Cabbage and Cilantro Salad

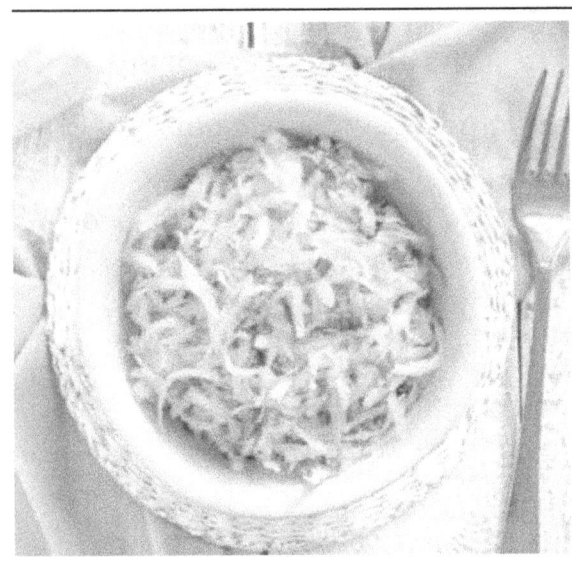

Cuba

Cuba is an island of the Caribbean. It has a rich history and culture.
The Cuban people are a mixture of Spanish, African, and indigenous heritage, and this is reflected in the island's music, food, and art. Cuba is known for its luxury cigars and rum.

INGREDIENTS

- Cabbage shredded ½ cup
- Red onion 1small
- Chopped cilantro ¼ cup
- Grated carrots 2
- Black pepper 1/4
- Oregano 1/4teaspoon
- Salt ¼ teaspoon
- Olive oil 1 teaspoon
- Lime juice 2 tab spoon
- Hot sauce
- Feta cheese

DIRECTIONS

1. Add chopped cilantro, red onions, shredded cabbage, grated carrot, olive oil, lime juice, hot sauce, salt, oregano, and crushed Black Pepper in a bowl. Mix until all well combined.
2. Serve and enjoy!

Dominican Republic: Beetroot Salad

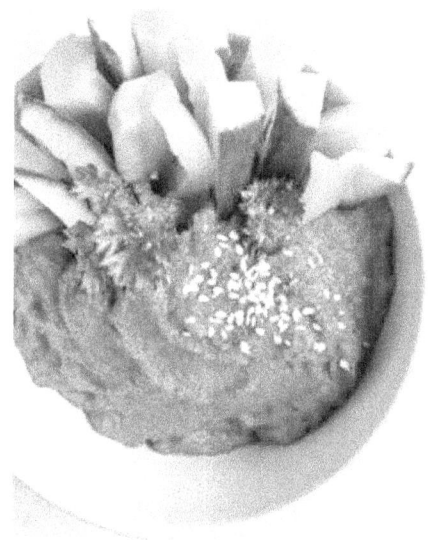

Dominican Republic

It is the 2nd largest country in the Caribbean and is home to some of the most beautiful beaches in the world.
The Dominican Republic is a favorite place of tourists. It is famous for its stunning scenery, its friendly people, and it's delicious food. Coffee is the national drink, and baseball is the national sport.

INGREDIENTS

- Boiled beetroot 1 cut into round slices.
- Tomato 1
- Cucumber 1 sliced.
- Red onions 1 cut into thin slices.
- Shredded cabbage 1 cup.

For dressing:

- Apple cider vinegar 4 tab spoon
- Olive oil or salad oil 2 tab spoon.
- Salt 1/2 teaspoon.

DIRECTIONS

1. Place all veggies in a bowl.
2. Mix dressing ingredients.
3. Drizzle over the salad veggies.
4. You can mix all vegetables or arrange all the Salads veggies in a serving plate and serve with dressing.

Haiti: Haitian Salad

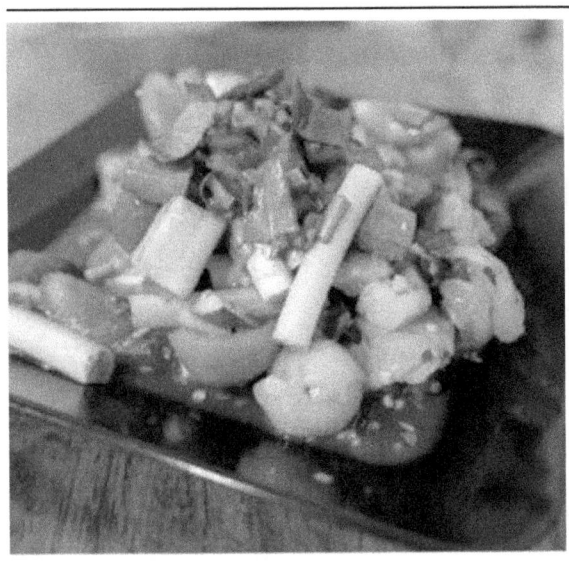

Haiti

Haiti is known as a piece of paradise in the Caribbean Sea that has the western third of the island of Hispaniola and some smaller islands like Gonâve, Tortue, Vache, and Grande Caye. The capital is Port-au-Prince. A place with historic monuments and blissful beaches.

Haiti's traditional dishes are Pikliz (tart with veggies), Diri ak djon djon (dish with soaked mushrooms), and Poulet aux noix (chicken with walnuts)

They mix fruit pulp with sugar and make cocktail juices named Jus grenadia and Cremas which is an alcoholic milk shake. Kokoye and Geele are the most popular beaches in Haiti and their zipline tour is never missed by tourists as it covers the crystal water and tropical view during the tour.

INGREDIENTS

- Chopped Watercress 1 bunch
- Red onion 1 small sized
- Garlic 1 clove
- Green bell pepper 1 sliced.
- Cucumber 2 thinly sliced.
- Avocado 1
- Olive oil ¼ cup
- Lime juice 2 tab spoon.
- Salt ¼ teaspoon
- Crushed black Pepper ¼

DIRECTIONS

1. Mix olive oil, vinegar, salt black pepper, and add all vegetables.
2. Toss well.
3. Scatter some radishes on top.

Guadeloupe: Green Salad

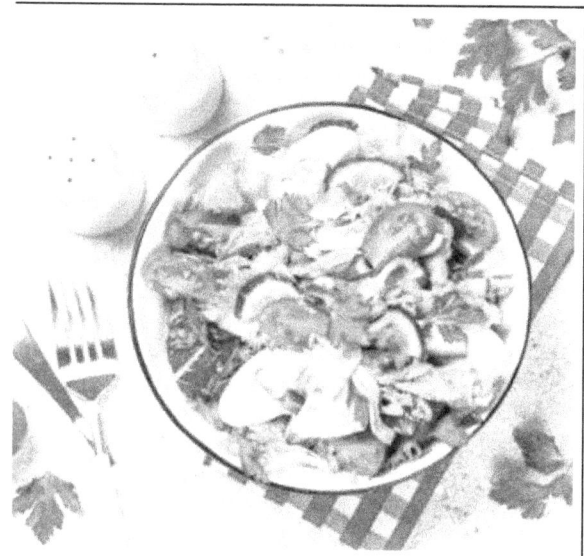

INGREDIENTS

- Mayonnaise 1/2 cup
- Sour cream 1/4 cup
- Lettuce
- White onion 1 chopped
- Carrot chopped 1
- Avocado 1
- Green bell pepper 1 julienne cut.
- Capers 2 tabspoon
- Fresh parsley or cilantro 2 tabspoon.
- Olive oil 2 tabspoon
- Hot sauce 2 tabspoon.
- Lemon juice 1 tabspoon
- Sugar 1 pinch
- Salt ¼ teaspoon
- Crushed black Pepper ¼ teaspoon.

Guadeloupe

Guadeloupe, an island in the Lesser Antilles, is a French territory with a rich culture and history.

The island is famous for its luxurious beaches in the Caribbean, cheese, butter, French wines and the fruit sauce.

During their months of carnivals, the whole archipelago get involves in dances on the cha-cha with the rhythms of drum and other instruments.

Guadeloupe is a popular tourist destination for history and beach lovers.

DIRECTIONS

1. Mix all ingredients until well combined.
2. Refrigerate for 1 hour and then serve.

Martinique : Parisian Salad

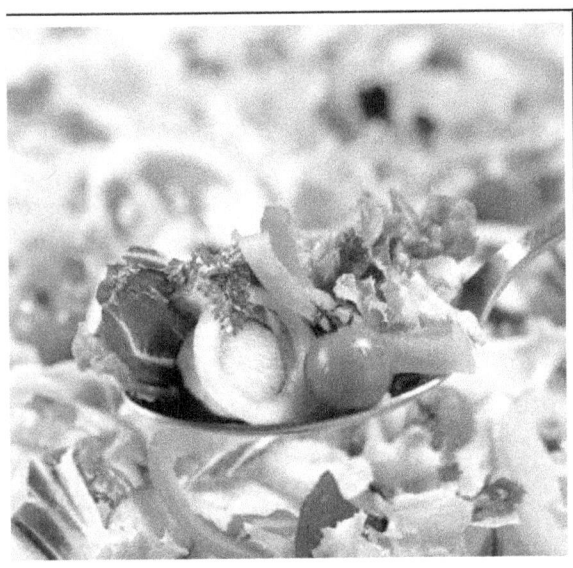

Martinique

Fort-de-France is the capital of the Martinique.

Their cultural heritage is presented through its intricate handicrafts and its delicious meals that are mixed with spices and mouth-watering flavors that will amaze your taste buds.

Including the island's many scents, cinnamon, vanilla, nutmeg and cloves of this region.

Martinique is known for the ideal conditions for sailing and windsurfing.

INGREDIENTS

- 1 small can of sweet corn, rinsed and drained
- 4 slices of ham cut into strips
- 100 g of Gruyere cheese, finely diced
- 2 tomatoes, diced
- 2 hard boiled eggs, sliced or quartered
- 6 Beautiful lettuce leaves

Ingredients for the Parisian Salad Sauce

- 1 teaspoon mustard
- 1 tablespoon of vinegar
- 3 tablespoons of vegetable oil
- 2 tablespoons of finely chopped parsley
- Salt & pepper

DIRECTIONS

1. Place the corn, slices of ham, tomatoes and cheese in a bowl. Mix.
2. Put mustard, vinegar, oil, parsley, salt and pepper in a jar with a lid. Seal and shake until the sauce is well emulsified. Pour the sauce over the salad and mix well.
3. Line a platter with the leaves of lettuce. Arrange the salad in the middle. Garnish the rim with slices of hard boiled eggs. Serve the salad, very fresh.

Indonesia: Indonesian Salad

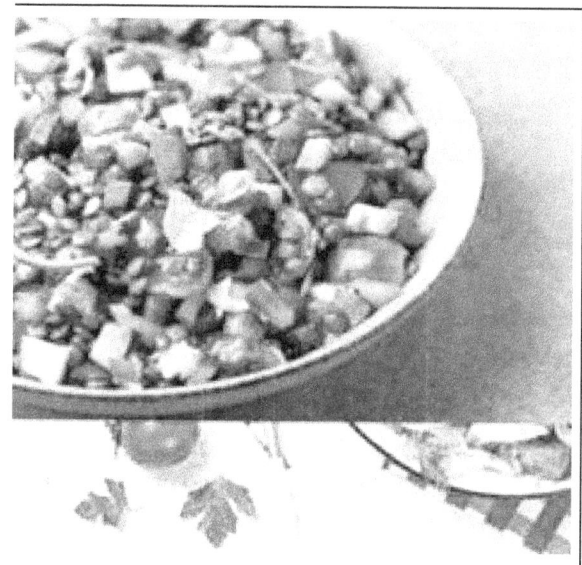

INGREDIENTS

- Grated coconut 1 cup
- Kaffir lime leaves 5
- Ginger
- Palm sugar
- Tamarind 1 teaspoon
- Dry Shrimp paste
- Garlic cloves 5
- Red chilies 3
- Onions 1
- Beans 1 cup.
- Spinach 1/2cup.
- Cabbage shredded 1 cup

Indonesia

Indonesia has around 17,000 islands and is the most popular place for surfing and cultural heritage.

The capital of Indonesia is Jakarta with beautiful artwork, people, cultures, customs, traditions, food, and landscapes.

Famous dishes in Indonesia include Nasi uduk, Sambar, fried rice, Satay (meat skewer), noodle soup and many more.

Egg drink, kopi joss (a kind of coffee), traditional soda, Wedang Jahe (ginger drink).

Tourists from all over the world visit Indonesia because of its beauty. Must go place are Ombak sunset, Masjid Agung, Les Villas, and Gili Islands.

DIRECTIONS

1. Blend onion, red chili, shrimp paste, garlic, and white turmeric
2. Heat 2 tab spoon oil, pour this mixture, and cook until the mixture gets fragrant.
3. Add kaffir lime leaves.
4. Add granulated or palm sugar
5. And cook until the sugar dissolve.
6. Add grated coconut and tamarind water and cook until all spices are well absorbed.
7. Then add cabbage, spinach, beans and cook for 5 minutes on low flame. Stir well.
8. Yummy Indonesian salad is ready to appease your taste bud

Myanmar: Burmese Cabbage Salad

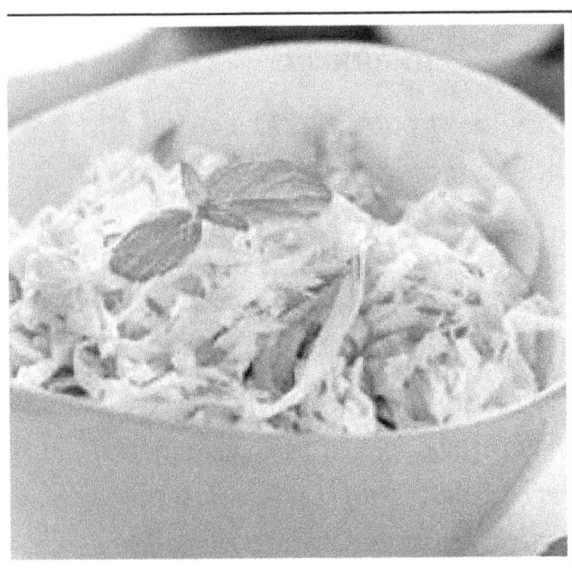

Myanmar

Myanmar / Burma is Southeast Asia country. Myanmar is bordered by Bangladesh, China, India, Laos, and Thailand.

Yangon is the country's largest city in Myanmar and is home to swarming markets, several parks and lakes. Naypyidaw is the capital city of Myanmar.

The country also boasts fabulous natural landscapes and lovely beaches.

Noodles is popular, especially their Mohinga fish curry, which is most loved by tourists, as well as their Mee Swan spicy noodles.

Bagan, the best way to take in this breathtaking city, take a hot air balloon and fly up in the air. The rides take place in the morning and one cannot leave this country without seeing this fascinating view.

INGREDIENTS

- Cabbage 1 and 1/2 cup
- Tomato 1 cut into slices
- Garlic chopped 1 teaspoon
- Cilantro chopped 1/4 cup
- Fish sauce 3 tab spoon
- Green chilies chopped 3 small
- Lemon juice 2 tab spoon.

DIRECTIONS

1. Add all veggies to a bowl.
2. Drizzle fish sauce, mix well and serve.

Vietnam: Vietnamese Salad

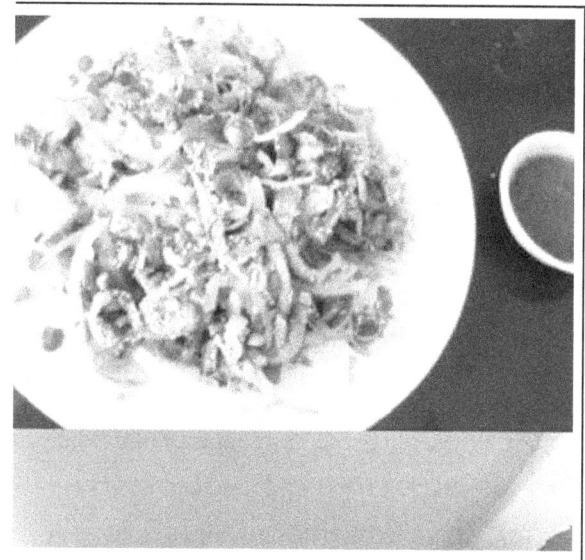

INGREDIENTS

- Cucumber 6 sliced
- Red onion 1 cut into rings
- Green onion green part only
- Salad Dressing Ingredients:
- Sesame oil 2 tab spoon
- Rice vinegar 2tab spoon Orange juice 1 tab spoon
- Crushed red chili 1 teaspoon
- Sugar 1 tab spoon
- Roasted sesame seeds 1 teaspoon

Vietnam

Vietnam is in the South China Sea. One of the world's best tourist destinations because of its calming beaches, tasty food, and culture. Vietnam is also famous for motorbikes, coffee, and crowded markets.

The food is well-known because of the use of fresh ingredients in dishes with many spices and herbs. Pho, Cha ca, Bot Chaien are some famous cuisines of Vietnam and their traditional drinks are soda herbal tea, fresh coconut water, and Bia.

This country is blessed with the largest cave in the world at Phong Nha-Ke Bang and French landmarks. Visitors can hardly enjoy them all in a single trip.

DIRECTIONS

1. Soak onion rings in hot water for 4 minutes.
2. Add cucumbers, red onions, and green onions to a bowl, pour dressing, and leave it for 5-10 minutes before serving.

China: Chinese Salad

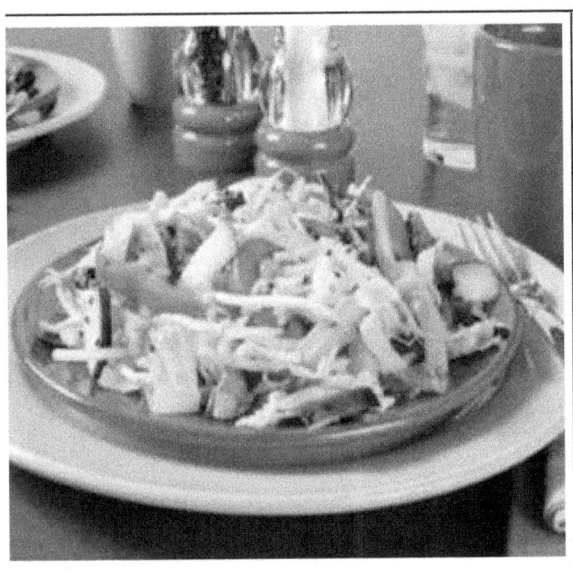

China

China is an East-Asian country with the capital city, Beijing. China is well known all over the world because of its best manufacturing techniques and trends. Some mouth-watering foods from China which are being eaten by all the countries of the world are Kung Pao Chicken, Sweet and Sour Pork, Hot Pot, Dim Sum, and Dumplings. The famous drinks that are preferred by tourists are plum drink, Boba milk tea, sweet rice wine, and Lychee wine.

The Great Wall of China, the Forbidden City, the Imperial Palace, Erhai Lake, and Summer Palace are the top rated tourist points of China.

INGREDIENTS

- Cabbage 1 cup shredded
- Celery 2 sticks
- Green onions 1/4 cup
- Soy sauce 2tabspoon
- Honey2tabspoon
- Vinegar 2 tab spoon
- Olive oil 2 tab spoon
- Roasted peanuts ¼ cup

DIRECTIONS

- Add all veggies to a bowl.
- Pour dressing, toss well and serve.

Australia: Australian Salad

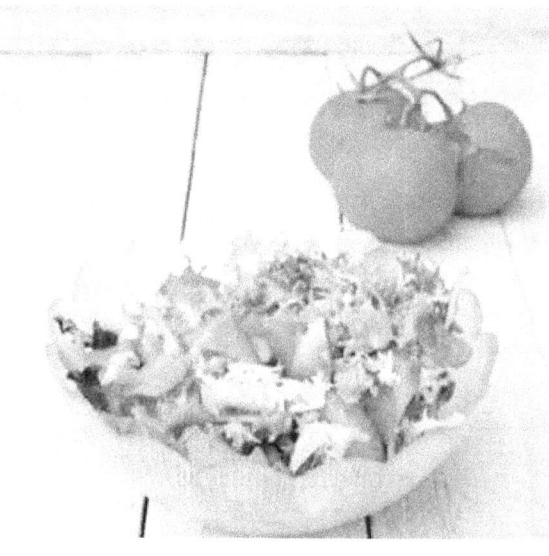

Australia

Australia, one of the largest countries in the world with capital of Canberra, a city that is well-known for museums and historical spots. Islands like Noosa, Bondi, Ningaloo reef, and Esperance are travelers' main visiting points in Australia.

Australian food never compromises on the quality of ingredients. Their main courses are with a combination of oysters as they are in an oceanic region and Australia also has the world's longest history in wine-making. Whisky, gin, rum and vodka are mixed with some additional flavors to enhance the national taste bud.

Kangaroo, Blue Mountains, and Litchfield National Park are fantastic sites for nature lovers.

INGREDIENTS

- Lettuce shredded 1 and 1/2 cup
- Tomatoes 2
- Cucumber 2 sliced
- Parsley 2 tab spoon
- Chives 2 tab spoon
- Baby spinach 1 cup roughly chopped
- Salt ¼ teaspoon
- Crushed Black Pepper 1/4 teaspoon.
- Red wine vinegar 2 tab spoon
- Olive oil 2 tabspoon
- Lime juice 2 tabspoon

DIRECTIONS

- Add lettuce, tomatoes, cucumber, baby spinach, parsley, and chives to a bowl.
- Mix olive oil, vinegar, lime juice, salt, black Pepper, and drizzle over the salad veggies.
- You have to serve this salad immediately for the best results.
- Mix all ingredients along with dressings before serving.

Kiribati: Kiribati Salad

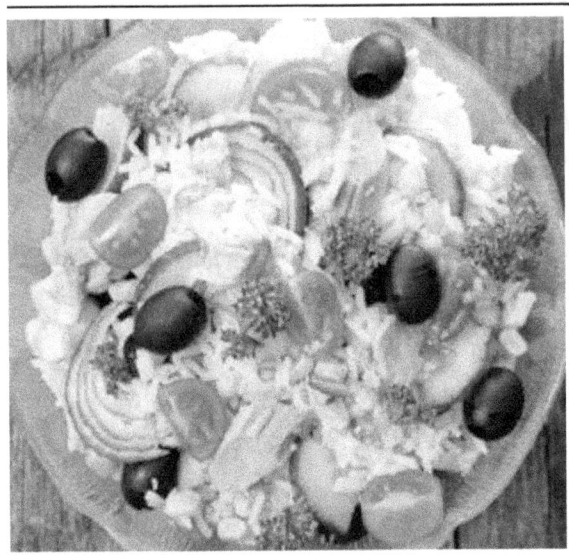

Kiribati

Kiribati is an island situated in the South Pacific Ocean. The name Kiribati comes from the Gilberts language and means "the end of the lines. The capital, Tarawa, has a population of just over 3,000 with world class fly-fishing, scuba diving, and outstanding seabird wildlife.

The Batata mash is a mixture of mashed potatoes with butter and coconut and their roasted lobster with coconut curry is really liked by visitors.

If you have a passion for exploring, discovering exotic places where few people have been before you will enjoy this place

INGREDIENTS

- Crab sticks 1 and 1/2cup
- Green onion 1 chopped
- Lettuce shredded 1 cup
- Tomato 1 chopped
- Corn 1 can
- Salt 1/4 teaspoon
- Crushed Black Pepper 1/4 teaspoon
- Mayonnaise ¼ cup
- Hard-boiled eggs 2
- Mozzarella 1/4 cup

DIRECTIONS

- Add crab sticks, lettuce, tomatoes, green onions, and chopped eggs to a bowl.
- Sprinkle salt and black Pepper.
- Add mayonnaise and toss well.
- Serve this salad on lettuce leave or chop them as I did. In both forms, the flavor comes out fine.

Micronesia: Micronesian Salad

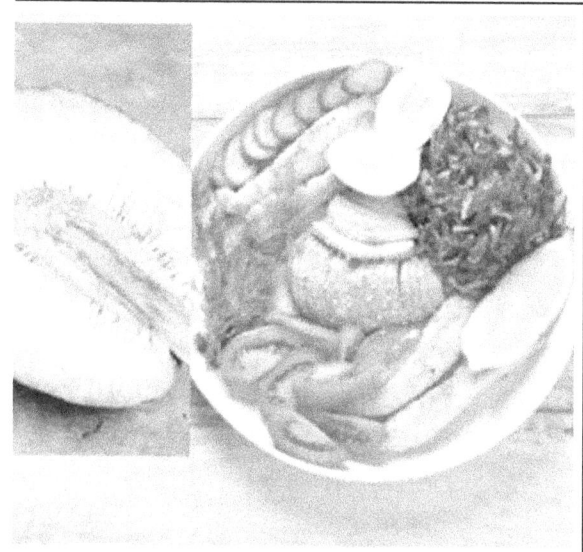

Micronesia

Micronesia is a located in the western Pacific Ocean. Its population is about 100,000 people. The capital city of Micronesia is Palikir with beautiful of waterfalls and forests. The main foods of Micronesia are yam, taro bread-fruit, and coconuts, with hundreds of varieties. Their ocean food is pelagic fish, shellfish, pigs, chicken, and crabs.

INGREDIENTS

- Boiled breadfruit 1
- Hard-boiled eggs 2
- Tomatoes 1 chopped
- Beans 1 cup boiled
- Cucumber 2 sliced
- Onions 1 chopped
- Dijon mustard 1/2 teaspoon
- Fried pork or chicken 1 cup
- Mayonnaise 1/4 cup
- Vinegar 2 tab spoon
- Sugar 1 pinch
- Salt 1/4 teaspoon
- Crushed Black Pepper 1/4 teaspoon.

DIRECTIONS

- Mix all veggies and chicken with mayonnaise in a bowl.
- Mix vinegar, Dijon mustard, salt, black Pepper and mix well
- Pour onto the salad.
- Chill for ½ hour and then serve.

Burkina Faso: Burkina Faso Salad

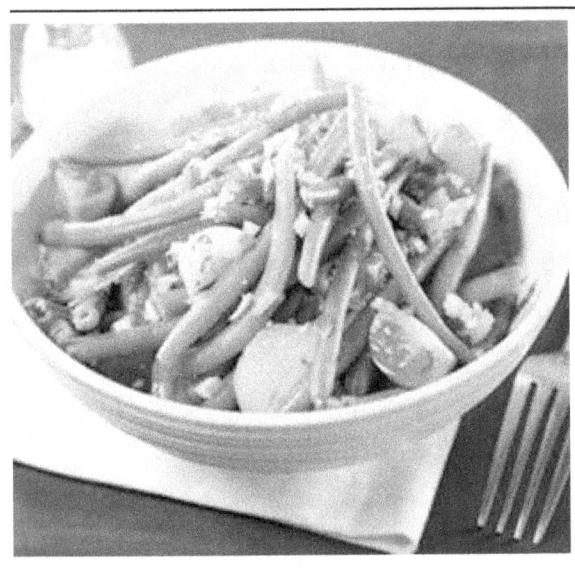

INGREDIENTS

- Green beans 250 g 2 and 1/2 cups
- White onion 1 small sized.
- Ginger chopped 1/2 teaspoon
- Garlic 1 teaspoon
- Red chili pepper 1
- Salt 1/2 teaspoon or to taste.
- Crushed black pepper 1/2 teaspoon.

Burkina Faso

Burkina Faso, bordered by Mali to the north, the Ivory Coast to the east, Niger to the southeast, and Burkina Faso and Ghana to the south. The capital and largest city is Ouagadougou.

Burkina Faso has about a 17 million population.

Burkina Faso is famous for its honest people, also known for pottery making and canvas art- work.

The main courses served are mutton, lamb, goat poultry, beef, and fish on a platter of veggies like tomato, zucchini, spinach, and onion.

Zoomkoom is the traditional drink, which is a mixture of pineapple with different spices. The parks, nature's life and wildlife visiting spots, and sculptures are popular places to enjoy.

DIRECTIONS

- Heat 2 tab spoon oil
- Add chopped onions, and cook until onions become soft and translucent.
- Add garlic, and satay until fragrant.
- Add red chili pepper, salt, black Pepper, and beans. Cook until beans are tender
- Serve hot.

Burundi: Burundian Salad

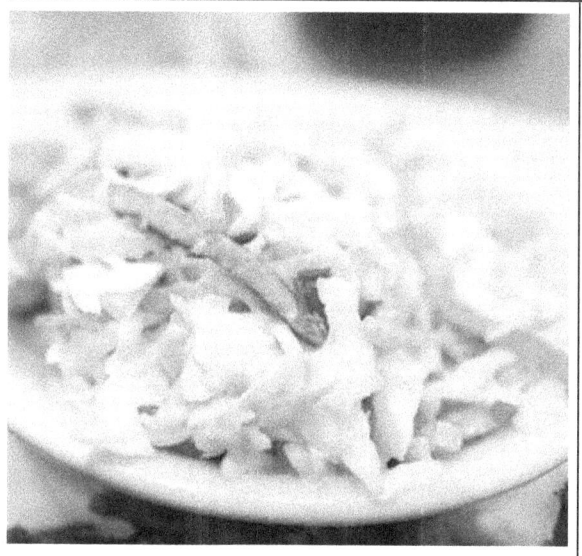

INGREDIENTS

- Cabbage shredded 1 and 1/2 cup
- Tomato 2 sliced
- Onion 1 chopped
- Cucumber 2 sliced
- Cabbage shredded 1 and 1/2 cup
- Tomato 2 sliced
- Onion 1 chopped
- Cucumber 2 sliced
- Red chili pepper chopped 1
- Salt 1/4 teaspoon
- Crushed Black Pepper 1/4 teaspoon
- Cilantro 1/4 cup chopped.
- Lemon juice 2 tab spoon.

Burundi

Burundi is located in the Great Lakes region of Central Africa.
The capital and largest city is Bujumbura.
The population of Burundi is estimated at just over 10 million.
Burundians enjoy a tradition of visual arts.
Flour porridge, curry, bean soup, and fried beans, are popular meals.
The drinks are the best combo of milk products with banana and cereal.
Landscapes of Burundi & the folk song dances are enjoyed by tourists.

DIRECTIONS

- Add cabbage, onion, tomato, red chili pepper .Season with some salt and black Pepper. Add lemon juice and toss all ingredients
- Add lemon juice and toss all ingredients.
- Chill for 1/2 hour before serving.

Egypt: Egyptian Salad

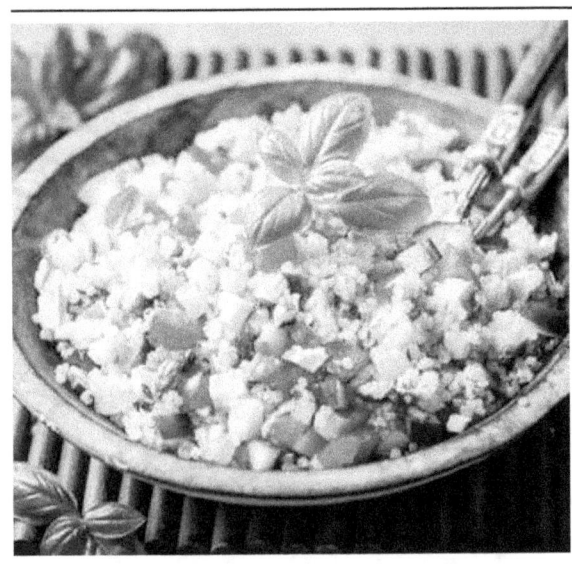

INGREDIENTS

- Tomatoes 2 diced
- Cucumbers 2 thinly sliced
- Carrots 1 chopped
- Red onions 1 chopped
- Fresh cilantro 1/4 cup chopped
- Parsley 2 tab spoon.
- Dill 2 tab spoon.
- For dressing water
- Vinegar 2 tab spoon
- Lemon juice 2 tab spoon
- Honey 1/2 teaspoon
- Water 1 cup
- Salt 1/4 teaspoon.
- Crushed Black pepper ¼ teaspoon
- Jalapeno 1 chopped
- Garlic crushed 1
- Ice or ice cubes as per your choice

Egypt

Egypt is one of the world's most complex and oldest cultures, and it has a rich history that goes back to before the beginning of recorded history.

The ancient Egyptians were advanced in their culture is renowned for its art, architecture, hieroglyphics and development of mathematics and science.

Shawarma is a popular dish cooked with grilled chicken, vegetables and sauces filled with pita bread.

The Museum of Egypt, Giza Necropolis, Siwa Oasis, Abu Simbel, and the River Nile Cruise are the main visiting places in Egypt

DIRECTIONS

- Add all dressing ingredients in a blender and blend well.
- Add all veggies to a bowl. Pour dressing water, cover, and chill for 1 hour for best results

Comoros: Comorian Salad

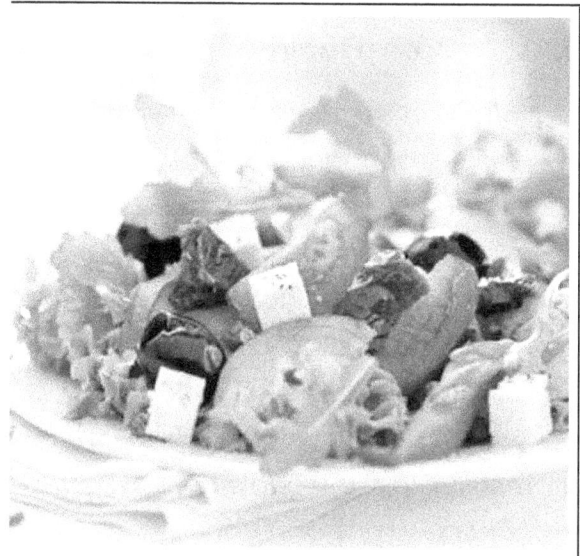

INGREDIENTS

- Lettuce iceberg thinly sliced wedges 1
- Tomato 1 halved.
- Capsicum 1 chopped.
- Radishes 1 or baby radishes 2 sliced
- Kalamata olives 1/2 cup.
- Shallot 1/2 cup chopped.
- Dill chopped 2 tab spoon.
- Olive oil 1/2 cup.
- Apple cider vinegar 2 tab spoon.
- Feta cheese crumbled 1/2 cup.
- Herbed Yogurt.
- Yogurt 1 and 1/2 cup.
- Lemon zest 1 teaspoon
- Lemon juice 2 tab spoon
- Garlic cloves chopped.
- Salt 1/4 teaspoon.

Comoros

The island nation of Comoros is a geographically small country located in the Indian Ocean. The population is approximately 1.3 million, and the capital is Moroni.

The islands are split into three main islands, Grande Comore, Anjouan, and Mohéli. The islands are popular tourist destinations for their beaches coral reefs, and its aromatic plants like vanilla and ylang-ylang. Pilaou (rice with meat and spices), boiled lobster in vanilla sauce, fish with coconut milk are mostly preferred by tourists. Drinks with coconut milk are traditional hits.

The best season to enjoy the Comoros is May till November, when the climate is moderate with rainfall.

DIRECTIONS

- Blend all herbed Yogurt ingredients and set aside.
- Set iceberg lettuce leaves on a serving platter.
- Pour olive oil and vinegar.
- Set tomato, capsicum, shallot, kalamata olives and radishes.
- Sprinkle some salt and black pepper.
- Add crumbled feta cheese.
- Garnish with chopped dill.
- Enjoy with herbed dressing.

Côte d'Ivoire: Cote d' Ivoire Salad

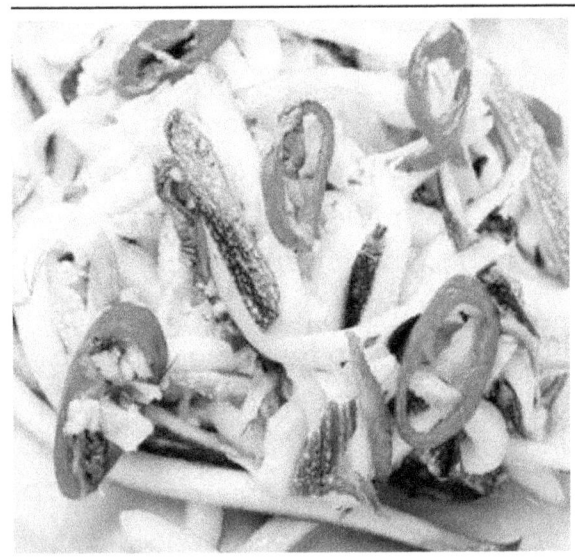

INGREDIENTS

- Courgetteszucchini 2 thinly sliced.
- Cucumbersthinly sliced 2
- Salt 1/4 teaspoon
- Crushed Black Pepper 1/2 teaspoon.
- Crushed red chili 1/2 teaspoon.
- White wine or apple cider vinegar 1 /2 cup
- Sugar 3 tab spoon
- Hot water half glass.

Côte d'Ivoire

Côte d'Ivoire is in the west of the African continent.
The country is bordered by Burkina Faso to the north and west, Ghana to the east, and Niger to the south.
The country has 22 million population. The official language of Côte d'Ivoire is French.
This is a country with lovely beach resorts and rainforests, also the world's best exporter of cashew nuts and cocoa.
They are best with plantains, yams, and cassava with vegetable sauce. Their traditional drinks are a mixture of ginger, orange juice and lime water

DIRECTIONS

- Mix vinegar, sugar, hot water, salt, and black Pepper in a bowl.
- Pour this dressing to all salad veggies.
- Leave it for 30 minutes, then serve this mouth-licking salad.

Newfoundland, Canada: Newfoundland Potato Salad

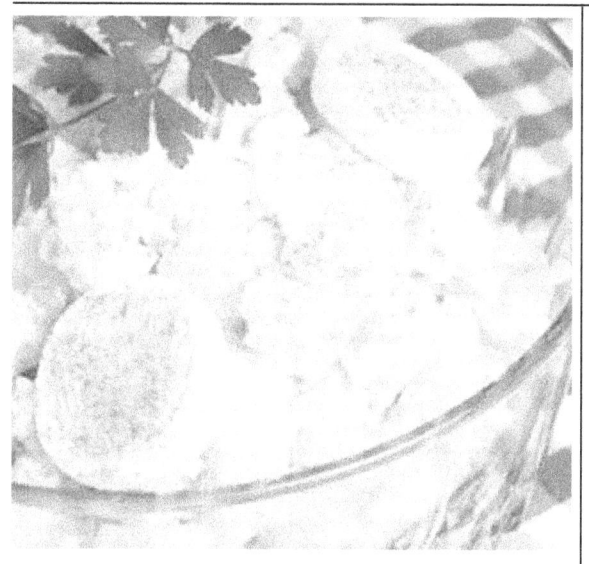

INGREDIENTS

- Potato boiled and chopped 3 medium-sized.
- Hard-boiled eggs 2
- Celery stalks 3
- Red onion 1 chopped
- Apple sliced 1
- Roasted Almonds 1/4 cup
- Mayonnaise 4 tab spoon.
- Mustard 1/2 cup.

Newfoundland, Canada

In Newfoundland and Labrador, you'll find rugged coastlines, vast wilderness, and abundant wildlife.
This province is home to the world's most northerly point, Cape Spear, and is also renowned for its stunning natural beauty. The capital city, St. John's, is known for its vibrant arts scene and beautiful architecture. Other provinces' major cities include Corner Brook, Placentia, and Grand Falls-Windsor. The province activities includes camping, climbing, and fishing in the late spring and snowshoeing, skiing, and snowmobiling in the colder time of year.
Their custom made stew, bunny pie, seal flipper, and wiener are popular food in Newfoundland.

DIRECTIONS

- Mix mayonnaise and mustard in a bowl. You can also add some salt and crushed Black Pepper to taste.
- Mix celery, apples, eggs, red onions, roasted almonds.
- Pour mustard mayo sauce
- Chill for 1/2hour and then serve

Los Cabos, Mexico: Special Salad

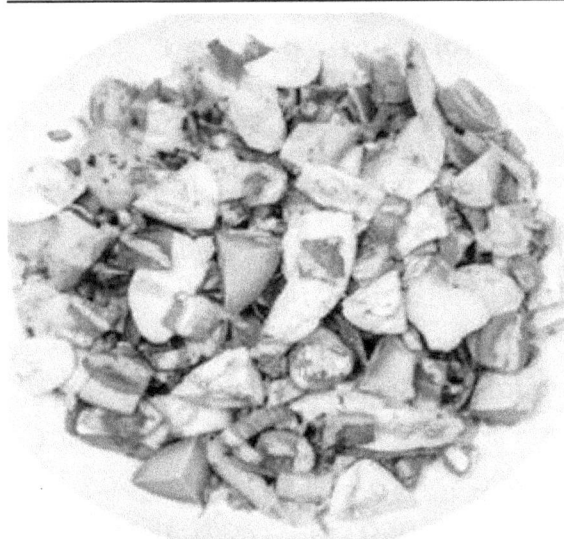

INGREDIENTS

- Cherry tomatoes 3 halved.
- Poblano chilies roasted
- Avocado 1 sliced
- Ear corns 2
- Feta cheese 1/2 cup crumbled
- Lemon juice 2 tabspoon
- Pepitas roasted 1 tabspoon.
- Caster sugar 1 pinch.
- Balsamic vinegar 1 tabspoon.
- Olive oil 2 tabspoon
- Fresh cilantro 1/4 cup
- Tortilla chips 1/4 cup

Los Cabos, Mexico

Los Cabos is in Baja, California, Mexico. The area has long been known for its stunning ocean, desert landscapes, dramatic cliffs, caves, and rock formations. Los Cabos has long been a popular tourist destination, with its dramatic cliffs and caves and dramatic ocean and desert landscapes. The area is also known for its luxury resorts and many activities, including golf, diving, fishing, horseback riding, and kayaking. Los Cabos is a great place to relax and enjoy the incredible scenery and activities available in the area. Los Cabos is located on the Baja California Peninsula in Mexico. Los Cabos is known for its clear waters, white-sand beaches, and lush vegetation.

DIRECTIONS

- Roast poblano chili in fry pan, cool, and set aside for later use.
- Mix all ingredients and serve.

Acapulco, Mexico: Acapulco Salad

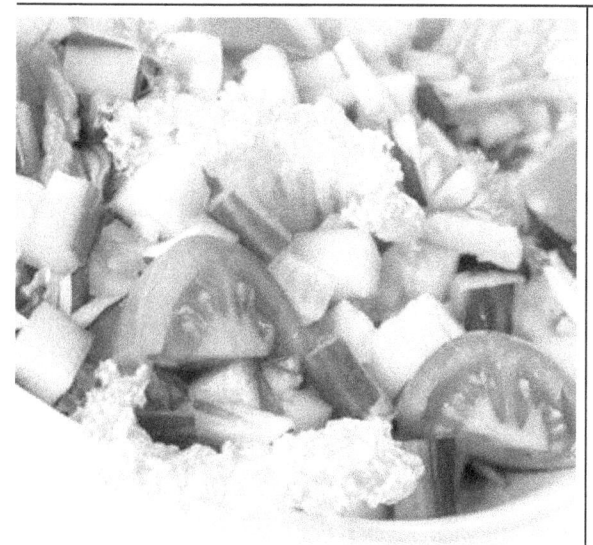

INGREDIENTS

- Lettuce chopped 1 cup
- Tomato 2 diced
- Cucumber 3 diced
- Green bell pepper thinly sliced.
- Fresh boiled peas 1/2 cup
- Green onion 1 chopped
- Pineapple cubes 1/4 cup
- Mayonnaise 1 cup
- Sour cream 1/4 cup
- Salt ¼ teaspoon
- Crushed Black Pepper 1/2 teaspoon

Acapulco, Mexico

Acapulco, Mexico, is best known as a hotspot for partying and luxury resorts.

There are also plenty of things to do in Acapulco aside from enjoying the nightlife. This city is packed with attractions, including some of Mexico's most famous landmarks.

There is also much more to explore in Acapulco if you're looking for a more relaxed experience.

The city has plenty of beaches, shopping, and restaurants, making it the perfect place to relax and recharge your batteries.

DIRECTIONS

- Mix mayo, sour cream, salt, black Pepper and set aside.
- Mix all veggies in mayo dressing and toss well.

Veracruz, Mexico: Veracruz Salad

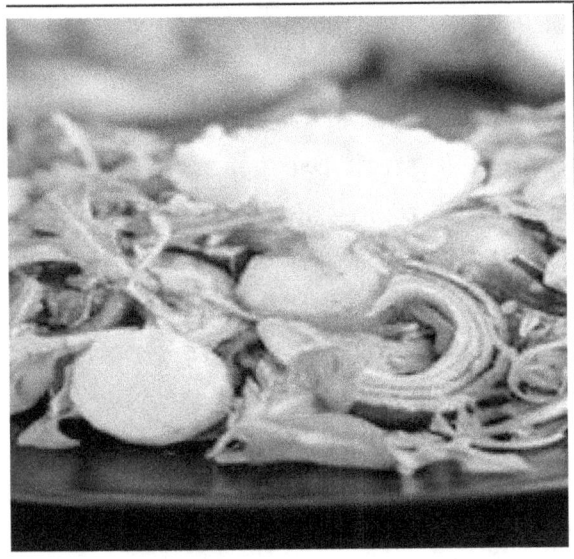

INGREDIENTS

- Lettuce 4 cups
- Tomatoes 2 cups chopped.
- Mexican potatoes, boiled, peeled, and cubed 1 cup.
- Corn chips 2 cups.
- Fresh cilantro 1/4 cup.
- Garlic minced 1 teaspoon
- Anchovy paste 1/2 teaspoon.
- Lemon or lime juice 4 tabspoon.
- Parmesan cheese ¼ cup.

Veracruz, Mexico

Veracruz, a state located in the south of Mexico, is one of the most popular tourist destinations in the country.

The state features a variety of landscapes and climates, making it a great place to visit year-round.

Veracruz is famous for its coral reefs and beautiful beaches.

The state has several popular tourist destinations, including Xalapa, the colonial city of Veracruz, and Manzanillo, the state's most important port.

Fascinating archaeological sites include the ancient city of Tula and the Templo Mayor, one of the largest pre-Columbian ruins in Mexico.

Veracruz is home to a variety of interesting cultures, including the Huasteca and Zapotec. The state is also home to several important musical traditions.

DIRECTIONS

- Mix parmesan cheese, fresh cilantro, lemon juice, anchovy paste, garlic, salt, and black Pepper.
- Add corn chips, Mexican potatoes, and lettuce and mix well.
- Garnish with some potato cubes and corn chips.

Boston, Massachusetts: Boston Salad

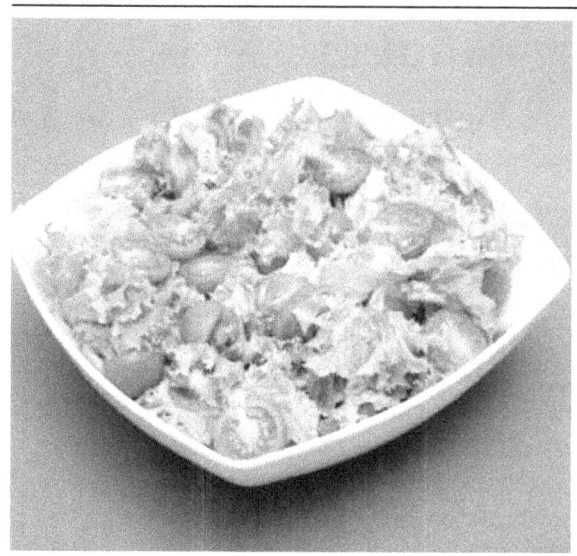

INGREDIENTS

- Boston lettuce 1 cup
- Roasted walnuts chopped 1/4 cup.
- Radishes 2 thinly sliced.
- Scallion 4 thinly sliced.
- Lemon juice 2 tab spoon.
- Olive oil or salad oil 2 tab spoon.
- White vinegar 2 tab spoon.
- Salt ¼ teaspoon
- Crushed Black Pepper 1/2 teaspoon

Boston, Massachusetts

Boston, Massachusetts, is a historic city located in the northeastern United States. With over 600 years of history, Boston is home to some of the country's oldest and most famous landmarks, such as the Freedom Trail and the USS Constitution Museum.

The city is also home to some of the most popular tourist destinations in the United States, including Fenway Park, the Boston Tea Party Museum, and the USS Constitution Museum.

DIRECTIONS

- Mix the vinegar, lemon juice, olive oil, salt, and crushed black Pepper in a bowl.
- Add the radishes, scallions, lettuce, fresh cilantro, scallions, and walnuts, and mix well.
- Top with some chopped walnuts.

St Louis, Missouri: Vegetable Salad

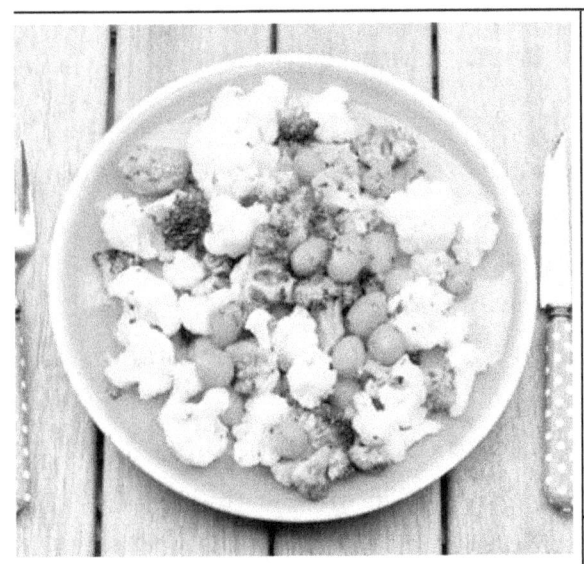

St Louis, Missouri

St Louis is a great city to live in! With a variety of attractions and events to choose from, there is always something to do. The city is home to the worldfamous Gateway Arch and the St. Louis Zoo and is also close to many other great attractions. The city has a variety of museums, parks, and historical sites to explore.

INGREDIENTS

- Cauliflower floret 2 cups
- Fresh broccoli 2 cups
- Red onion 1 chopped
- Parmesan cheese 1/4 cup
- Salt 1/4 teaspoon.
- Crushed Black Pepper 1/2 teaspoon
- Mayonnaise 1 cup
- Sugar 3 tab spoon
- Honey 1/2 teaspoon.
- Becan or ham fried and crumbled 4

DIRECTIONS

- Mix mayonnaise, cheese, honey, sugar, salt, pepper.
- Add broccoli, cauliflower florets, red onions,
- Pour dressing over vegetables.
- Serve and enjoy this yum salad!

Italy: Italian Salad

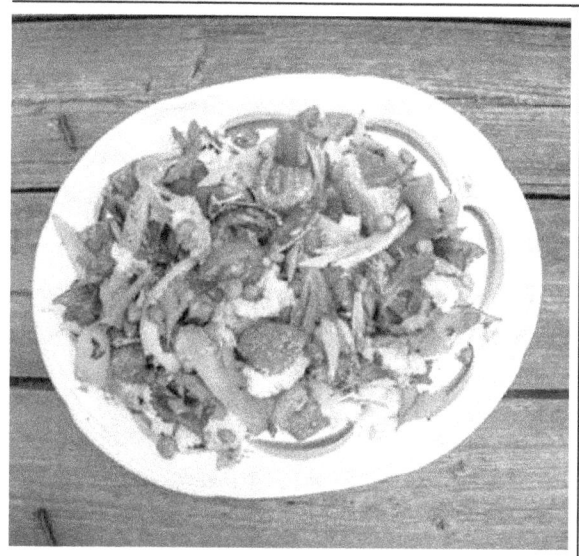

INGREDIENTS

- Tomatoes 2 medium-sized
- Cucumber 1 diced
- Fresh chopped parsley 1/4 cup.
- Green onions green part only 3
- Fresh mint chopped 2 tab spoon.
- Olive oil 4 tab spoon.
- Lemon juice 2 tab spoon
- Salt ¼ teaspoon.
- Crushed Black Pepper 1/4 teaspoon or to taste.

Italy

Italy is in Southern Europe. Italy is renowned for its travel industry, Rome is the capital of Italy and quite possibly one of the most renowned cities in the nation. Italy is known for its language, drama, design and its extravagant brands. Renowned food varieties of this famous nation are pizzas, tiramisu, espresso, and Italian salads. Italy has been home to numerous civilizations. The leaning tower of Pisa is perhaps the most renowned landmark in Italy and Venice (the city on water) is additionally the most appealing sight for travelers.

DIRECTIONS

- Mix All Veggies
- Mix All Dressing Ingredients and Drizzle On Mixed Veggies.
- And Enjoy!

Andorra: Chicory Salad

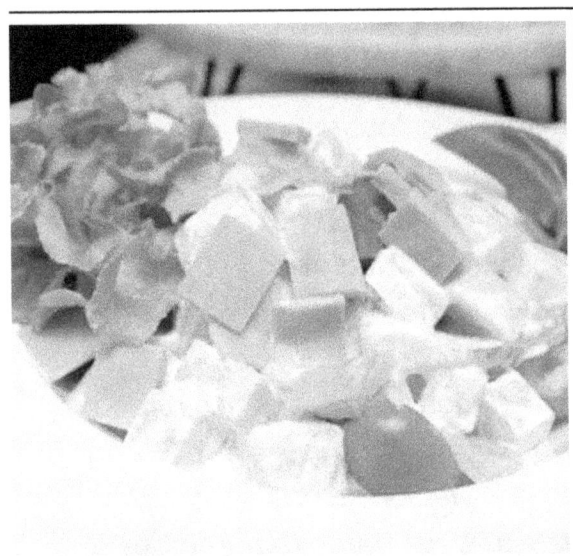

Andorra

Andorra is a small landlocked country situated in the Pyrenees Mountains between France and Spain.

Andorra is known for its high mountain ranges, such as the Pyrenees and the Pre-Pyrenees, its ski resorts, its luxury goods. Andorra is known as a famous traveler's place, the next time you are there check out the mountainous ranges, zip lines, and ski slopes.

INGREDIENTS

- Chicory green ½ bunch
- Crushed garlic 1 teaspoon.
- Ham or fried bacon 1 cup crumbled
- Olive oil 2 tab spoon
- Apple cider vinegar 2 tab spoon.
- Salt ¼ teaspoon.
- Crushed Black Pepper 1/4 teaspoon.

DIRECTIONS

- Soak green chicory in water for 2 hours.
- Wash chicory, add olive oil, vinegar, salt, black Pepper, chopped garlic, fried crumbled bacon, and mix well.

Liechtenstein: Liechtenstein Salad

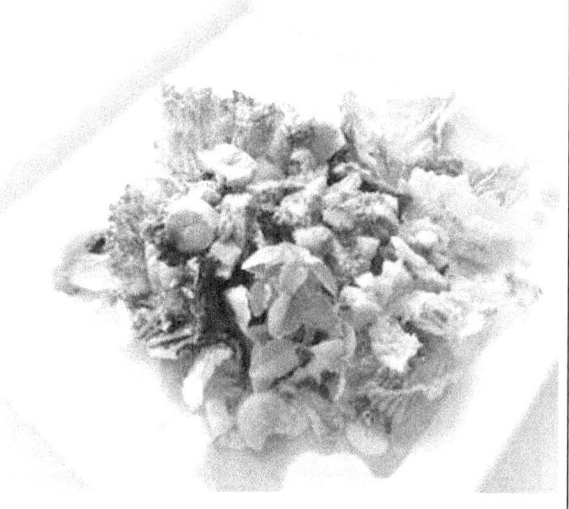

INGREDIENTS

- Lettuce leaves 3
- Cooked lobster meat sliced 1 cup.
- Mushrooms sliced 1/4 cup.
- Red onion 1 chopped.
- Butter 1 tab spoon
- Salt 1 /2 teaspoon.
- Crushed black pepper 1/4 teaspoon.
- Paprika powder 1/2 teaspoon
- Whipped cream 1 cup.
- Olive oil 2 tab spoon
- Lemon juice 2 tab spoon.
- Mustard powder 1/2 teaspoon.

Andorra

Andorra is a small landlocked country situated in the Pyrenees Mountains between France and Spain.

Andorra is known for its high mountain ranges, such as the Pyrenees and the Pre-Pyrenees, its ski resorts, its luxury goods. Andorra is known as a famous traveler's place, the next time you are there check out the mountainous ranges, zip lines, and ski slopes.

DIRECTIONS

- Mix cream, olive oil, lemon juice, salt, pepper, and paprika.
- Melt butter and satay mushrooms for a few seconds on medium flame.
- Add lobster meat, red onion, cream sauce, and toss well.
- Garnish with onion rings and some mushroom slices.

San Marino: San Marina Salad

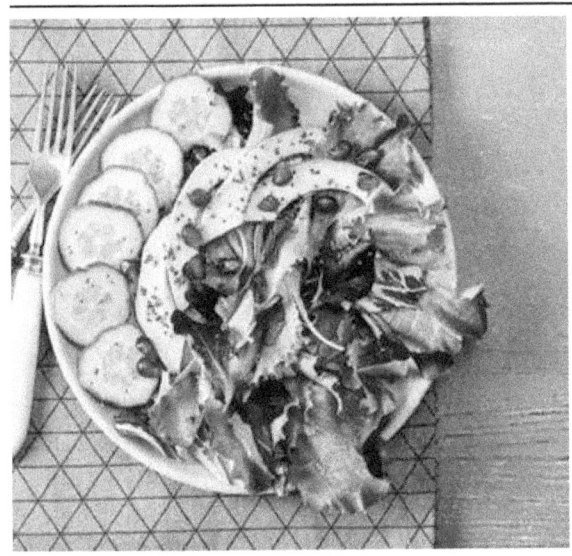

San Marino

San Marino is a small independent country located in the heart of Europe.
The country has a population of just over 33,000 and comprises six small towns and one capital city, San Marino.
The pizza, gelato ice cream, and pasta are Fantastic; the San Remo mixed drink as well as wine, cheese and handicraft.
Walks around the limited cobbled roads are thrilling for sightseers. San Marino Lake in Faetano is also famous for fishing.

INGREDIENTS

- Lettuce 2 leaves
- Avocado 1 sliced.
- Cucumber sliced 3
- Fried calamari tubes or corned tuna 1 cup.
- Salt 1 pinch
- Crushed Black Pepper 1/4 teaspoon
- Feta cheese crumble 1/4 cup

DIRECTIONS

- Set lettuce leaves onto a serving plate.
- Place Cucumber slices, avocado
- Add salt and Pepper. Add calamari tubes or corned tuna.
- Sprinkle crumbled feta cheese on top.

Holy See : Holy See Salad

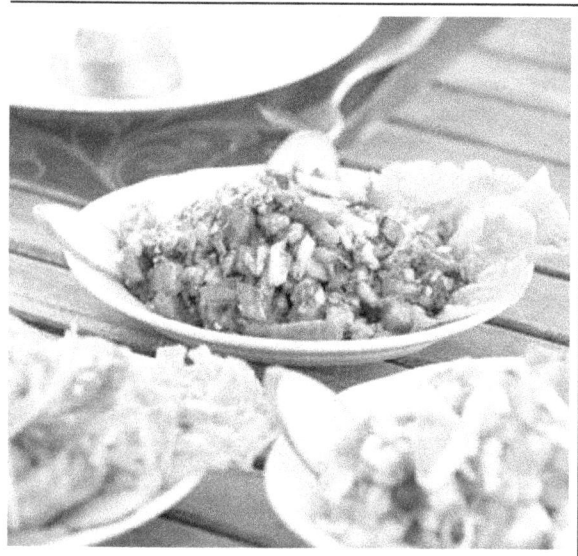

INGREDIENTS

- Tomatoes 2 chopped
- Red onions 1 chopped
- Cucumber 2 sliced
- Red chili pepper 2 chopped
- Walnut 2 tab spoon.
- Garlic 1

Holy See

The Holy See is frequently referred to by the term the Vatican, situated in the city of Rome in Italy.
The climate is moderate with precipitation and dry during summers.
Check out the panoramic view of St Peter's square, the Vatican Secret Archives. Parmesan, Scappi's Brocolli, Cato's cheddar bread, tiramisu, espresso, and unadulterated wines are some mouth-watering and invigorating delights of the Holy See

DIRECTIONS

- Blend mayonnaise, garlic, almonds, water, vinegar, salt, and Pepper.
- Mix all veggies.
- Serve this dressing with salad.

Section 11

Vegetable Salads

Panama: Panama Salad

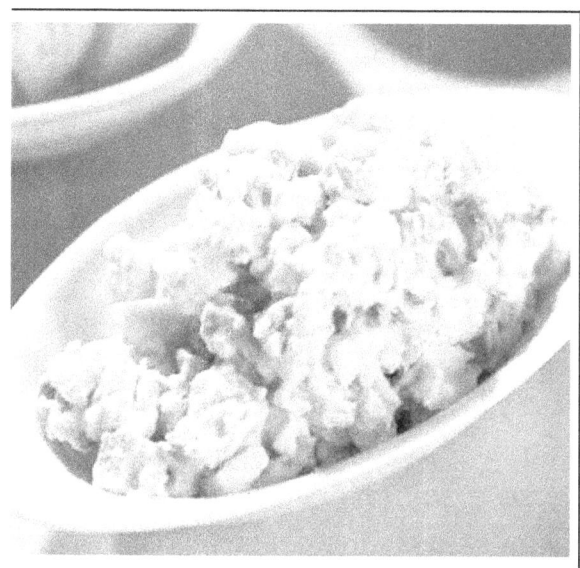

Panama

The Panama Canal is a sea route connecting the Pacific and Atlantic Oceans.
It is the only route between the two oceans in Central America.
The Panama Canal is also one of the most important trade routes in the world.
Construction of the Panama Canal began in 1904 and was completed in 1914
Rice, Corn meat and vegetables are popular dishes.
Enjoy the mountains, tropical jungles, wonderful white-sand sea shores fill with interesting animals, flowers, and tree species.

INGREDIENTS

- Boiled potatoes 2 cut into cubes.
- Boiled beets 2 cubes
- Hard-boiled eggs 2
- Spring onion 1 chopped.
- Salt 1 /4 teaspoon
- Black Pepper 1/4 teaspoon
- Mayonnaise 1/2 cup.

DIRECTIONS

- Mix all veggies in a bowl.
- season with some salt and Pepper.
- Add mayonnaise and toss well

Costa Rica: Costa Rican Salad

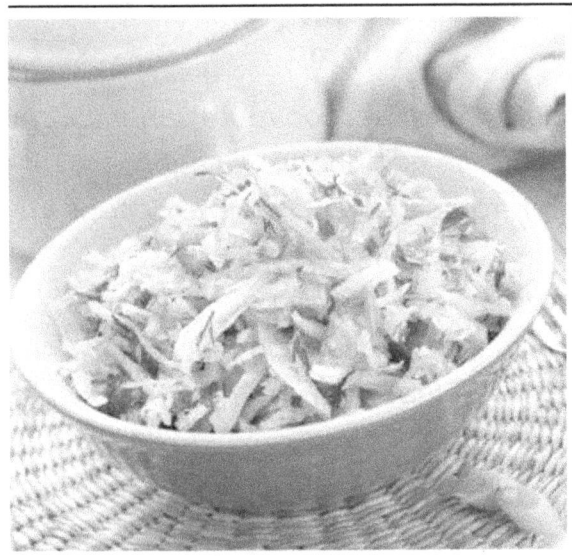

INGREDIENTS

- Cabbage thinly sliced 4 cups.
- Fresh cilantro 1/2 cup
- Lime juice 2 tab spoon
- Olive oil 2 tab spoon
- Salt 1/4 teaspoon
- Black Pepper 1/4 teaspoon
- For Garnishing.
- Parsley 2 tab spoon
- Spring onion (optional)

Costa Rica

Costa Rican nature is a paradise for nature lovers.
The country is rich in biodiversity and home to a wide variety of plants and animals. Costa Rica is also known for its pristine beaches and clear waters.
The country is home to some of the world's most beautiful volcanoes and rainforests. Costa Rica is a great destination for travelers who want to enjoy the country's natural beauty without any hassle.

DIRECTIONS

- Mix cilantro, cabbage, olive oil, lime juice, salt, and Pepper.
- Garnish with some parsley, lemon wedge, and spring onion

Chile: Chilean Salad

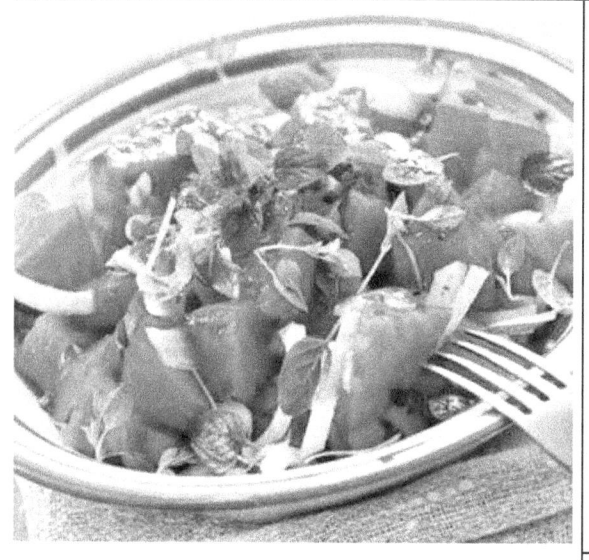

Chile

Chile is a beautiful country with a rich cultural heritage.
Chile is home to the Atacama Desert, which is the driest place on Earth, with the world's largest salt flat.
Chile is also home to the Andes, the tallest mountains in the world.
It is a great place to visit for its beautiful scenery and diverse culture.

INGREDIENTS

- Onion 1 cut into rings
- Tomato 1 sliced
- Fresh cilantro ¼ cup
- Lime juice 4 tab spoon
- Olive oil 2 tab spoon.
- Salt ¼ teaspoon
- Crushed black pepper ¼ teaspoon

DIRECTIONS

- Soak onion slices in hot water for 5 minutes.
- Mix tomato, soaked onion slices, cilantro, lime juice, salt, Pepper, and olive oil in a bowl.
- Garnish with some chopped cilantro.

Colombia: Columbian Salad

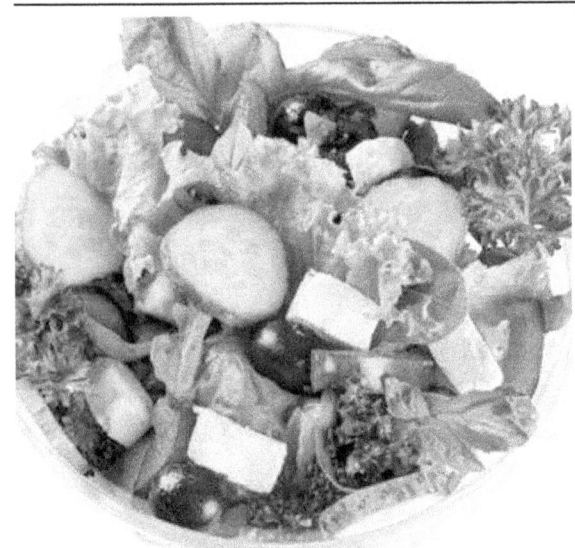

Colombia

Colombia is the most bio-diverse country in the world.
It is also home to one of the world's largest natural gas reserves and to a number of indigenous groups, including the Achiari, the Wayuu, and the Kogi.
Pandebono Colombiano, Fritanga (Grill), and Arepas are some popular Colombian foods. Guaro is the sweet beverage.

INGREDIENTS

- Olive oil 1/2 cup.
- Garlic chopped 1 teaspoon.
- Vinegar 2tabspoon
- Oregano 1 teaspoon.
- Salt ¼ teaspoon
- Black pepper ¼ teaspoon
- For salad
- Chopped lettuce 4 cups
- Onion 1 sliced
- Tomato 1 sliced
- Green olives 10
- Parmesan cheese 1/4 cup.
- Swiss cheese 1/4cup
- Lime or lemon juice 2 tabspoon
- Ham slices 6

DIRECTIONS

- Mix olive oil, garlic, vinegar, lime juice, oregano, salt, and black Pepper.
- Mix lettuce, ham, slices, tomato, onion, green olives, Swiss cheese
- Pour dressing to all mixed veggies and Swiss cheese.
- Sprinkle parmesan cheese and squeeze lemon juice when you serve this salad.

Ecuador: Ecuadorian Salad

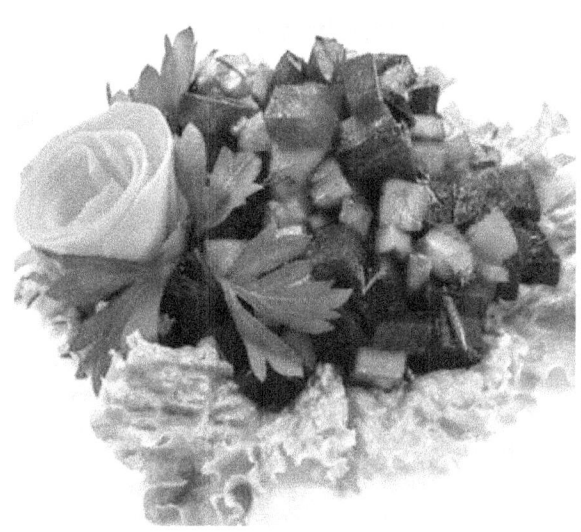

INGREDIENTS

- Boiled carrots 2
- Boiled beets 1
- Lettuce chopped 1 cup
- Green onions 2 green part only.
- Parsley 2 tabspoon.
- Lemon juice of 1 lemon.

Ecuador

Ecuador is a located in the south-western corner of South America.

Colombia borders it to the south and southeast, Peru to the east, and the Pacific Ocean to the west.

The country has an area of approximately 297,000 square kilometers, making it the smallest country in South America.

Canelazo drink is popular for cold and rainy evenings and a popular dish is Bolon de Verde (balls made of green banana with cheddar).

The capital city of Ecuador is Quito. The country is well known for its varied natural attractions, including the Galápagos Islands, the Amazon Rainforest, the Andes, and the Sierra Nevada.

DIRECTIONS

- Mix carrots, beets, green onions. Sprinkle salt, Pepper, and squeeze lemon juice
- Top with some green onion.

Puerto Rico: Puerto Rico Salad

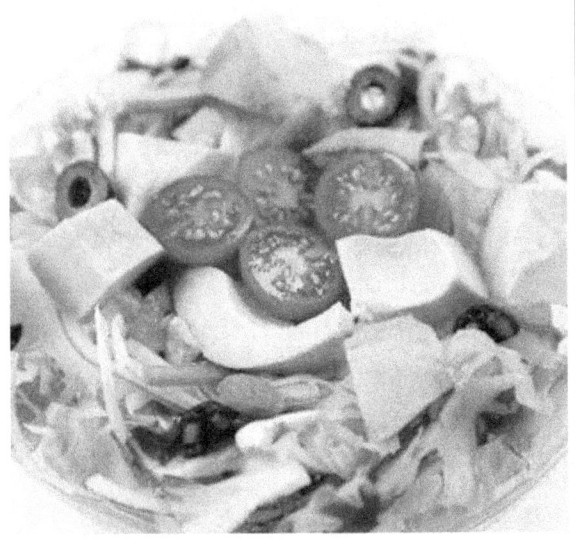

Puerto Rico

The island is in the Caribbean Sea, southeast of the U.S. Virgin Islands and northwest of the Dominican Republic.

The capital city is San Juan. Arepas de Maiz, Barriguitas de Viejas, and kidney stew are famous dishes.

Popular beverages includes coconut milk and cocoa.

From delightful sea shores to regular tropical jungles, Puerto Rico has interesting attractions to keep coming back.

INGREDIENTS

- Sweet potatoes boiled and cubed 2
- Avocado 1 sliced
- Pumpkin boiled or steamed 1 cut into slices
- Green onions 1 sliced.
- For dressing.
- Lime juice 2 tabspoon
- Olive oil 2 tabspoon
- Honey 1/2 teaspoon.
- Salt 1/4 teaspoon
- Black Pepper 1/4 teaspoon.
- Lettuce leaves 2-3

DIRECTIONS

- Mix sweet potato, avocado, and green onion.
- Mix dressing ingredients.
- Pour dressing onto the mixed veggies.
- Chill for 1 hour before dinner or any meal of your choice.

Saint-Barthélemy: Saint-Barthélemy Salad

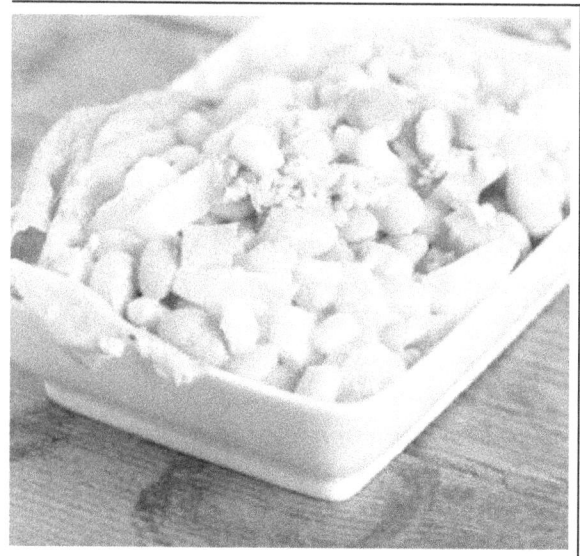

INGREDIENTS

- Whole kernel corn 1 and 1/2 cup from can
- Red bell pepper 1 chopped
- Green onion 1 chopped
- Tomato 2 chopped.
- Cucumber 1 thinly sliced.
- Jalapeno 1 chopped.
- Dill 2 tabspoon.
- Fresh parsley 2 tabspoon.
- For dressing
- Olive oil 2 tabspoon.
- Lemon juice 2 tabspoon.
- Honey or sugar 1/2 teaspoon.
- Salt 1/4 teaspoon
- Crushed black pepper 1/4 teaspoon.

Saint-Barthélemy

Saint-Barthélemy is an island in the Caribbean Sea, part of the Kingdom of France.

The island is known for its natural beauty, including its calm waters, white-sand beaches, and lush vegetation.

Saint-Barthélemy is also known for its rich history, including its role in the development of Christopher Columbus's exploration of the Americas.

Today, Saint-Barthélemy is a popular tourist destination, with many visitors coming to enjoy its natural beauty and history.

DIRECTIONS

- Mix all dressing ingredients.
- Add all salad veggies, pour dressing, and toss well.
- Serve chill for best results.

Saint-Martin: Saint Martin Salad

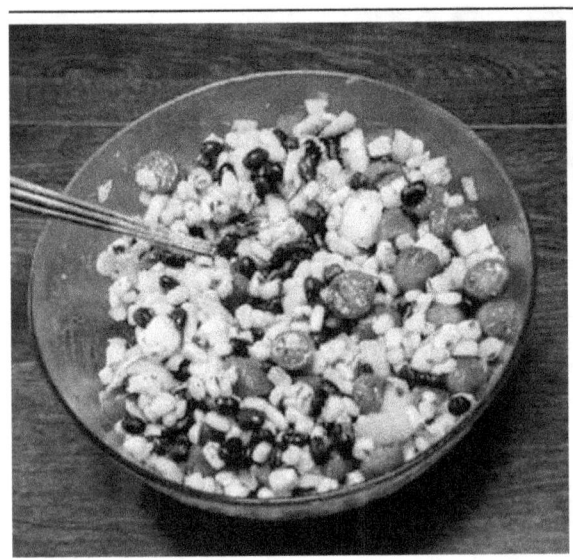

Saint-Martin

Saint-Martin is an island in the Caribbean Sea.

Saint-Martin, which is divided into two parts, the French side, and the Dutch side, is about 120 kilometers long and 50 kilometers wide.

The population of Saint-Martin is about 40,000.

The official language of Saint-Martin is French, but Dutch is also spoken.

Saint-Martin is known for its beautiful beaches, turquoise waters, lush tropical forest and luxury resorts.

INGREDIENTS

- Tomato 2 chopped
- Green bell pepper 1 thinly sliced
- Cucumber 1 thinly sliced
- Sweet corn 1/2 cup.
- Jalapeno 1 chopped
- Fresh parsley chopped 1/2 cup
- Olive oil 2 tab spoon
- Lemon juice 1 tab spoon
- Salt 1/4 teaspoon.
- Crushed Black Pepper 1/4 teaspoon.

DIRECTIONS

- Mix tomatoes, cucumbers, green bell pepper, fresh parsley, sweet corn, jalapenos,
- Add dressing ingredients and mix well again.

Jamaica: Jamaican Salad

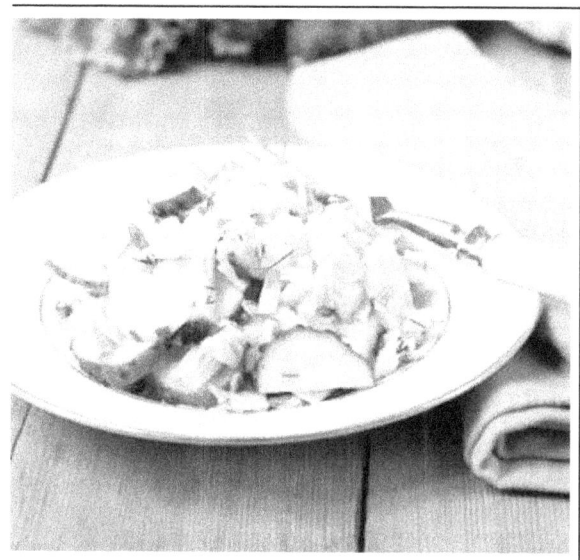

Jamaica

Jamaica is a Caribbean Island with its capital in Kingston.
It is known or it popular tourist attractions in Montego Bay and Negril.
Jamaica is home to reggae music, Bob Marley, great food and it popular sports are Track & Field, Soccer and Cricket.
The people of Jamaica are friendly and hospitable. The jerk, curry, pepper pot soup, Red Stripe beer, and Blue Mountain coffee are the best hits for travelers.

INGREDIENTS

- Cabbage shredded 1 cup
- Cucumber 2 diced
- Tomato 2 sliced
- Cherry tomato 2
- Sweet corn 1/2 cup
- Salt 1/4 teaspoon
- Black Pepper 1/4 teaspoon

DIRECTIONS

- Mix all veggies Sprinkle salt, Pepper, and toss well.

Trinidad & Tobago: Trinidadian Potato Salad

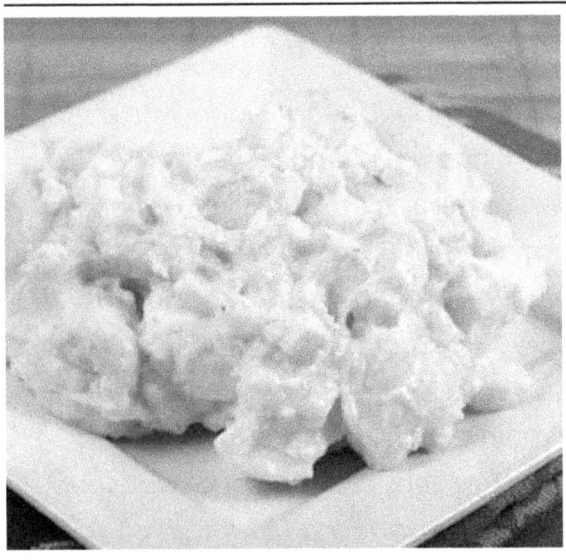

Trinidad & Tobago

It's a Caribbean Island sharing maritime borders with Guyana
Trinidad is the country's largest and most populous island, while Tobago is the smallest. Trinidad and Tobago are twin island countries separated by a narrow strait. The islands are known for their calypso music, carnival celebrations,& steel pan. Exotic curry & roti, sea food, dumplings, yams, stews, mauby, sorrel, and sea moss will enhance your taste buds.

INGREDIENTS

- Boiled and cubed potatoes 5 medium-sized.
- Garlic 2 cloves chopped.
- Red chili pepper 4
- Green onion 2 chopped
- Celery 1 stick
- Garlic crushed 1 teaspoon
- Mix vegetables (peas, sweet corn, carrot, bell pepper) 1 cup
- For mayo dressing
- Mayonnaise 1 cup.
- Mustard 1/2 teaspoon.
- Salt 1 teaspoon
- Black Pepper 1/4 teaspoon.
- Vinegar 2 tabspoon
- Lemon juice 2 tabspoon
- Brown sugar 1 tabspoon.
- Hot water 2 tabspoon.

DIRECTIONS

- Mix all salad ingredients.
- Mix mayo, mustard, salt, black Pepper, vinegar, lemon juice, brown sugar, and hot water. The dressing is ready.
- Mix mayo dressing in salad ingredients well.
- Refrigerate for 1/2 hour and then serve.

Mongolia: Mongolian salad

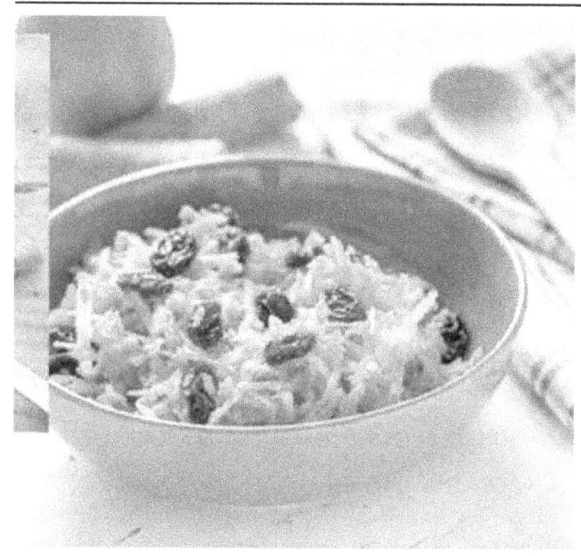

INGREDIENTS

- Carrots Julienne cut 2 cups.
- Raisins or black currents 1/2 cup
- Soak in hot water for 1/2 hour.
- For Mongolian dressing
- Oil 2 tab spoon
- Lemon juice 3 tab spoon.
- Salt 1 pinch
- Black Pepper 1/4 teaspoon.
- Sugar 1 teaspoon.

Mongolia

Mongolia is an amazing country. It's vast and diverse, with many different types of weather. The landscape is gorgeous, with mountains, valleys, steppes, and deserts.
The people are loving, friendly, and hospitable, and the culture is fascinating. Mongolia is known for the Blue Skies, two hump camels &
its nomadic people living traditional lives, moving around the country with their animals.
They are skilled at horseback and camel riding, archery and wrestling.
Feast upon the stuffed dumplings and conventional wine blended in with milk- Ayrag.

DIRECTIONS

- Mix dressing ingredients.
- Add carrots, raisins and mix all until well combined.
- Refrigerate for 1 hour, and then serve

Armenia: Armenian Salad

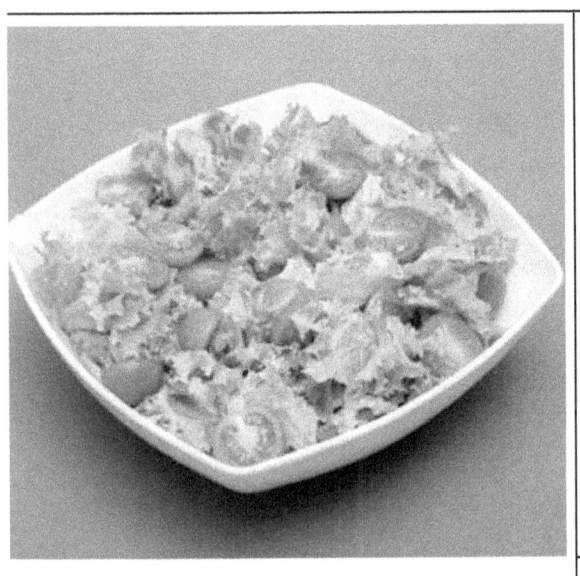

Armenia

Armenia is in the eastern Caucasus, bordering Azerbaijan and Turkey. The region is mountainous and has a temperate climate.
The capital is Yerevan.
Armenia is home to over 3 million people. The national food is Delma served with vine and Cognac an alcoholic drink, made with special grape extract.

INGREDIENTS

- Romaine lettuce chopped 1 cup
- Tomato 1 sliced
- Red onion 1 chopped.
- Cucumber 1 sliced.
- Red bell pepper 1 thinly sliced.
- Olives 1/2 cup sliced.
- Fresh mint chopped 2 tabspoon.
- Feta cheese crumbled 1/4 cup.
- Dressing ingredients.
- Olive oil 1/4 cup.
- Lemon juice 2 tabspoon.
- Sugar 1 pinch.
- Dried mint 1 teaspoon.
- Salt 1/4 teaspoon.
- Crushed Black Pepper 1/4 teaspoon.

DIRECTIONS

- Whisk together all the dressing ingredients.
- In a large bowl, mix all salad vegetables.
- Drizzle dressing over this Armenian salad.
- Mix well and enjoy!

Asia

Azerbaijan: Azerbaijan salad

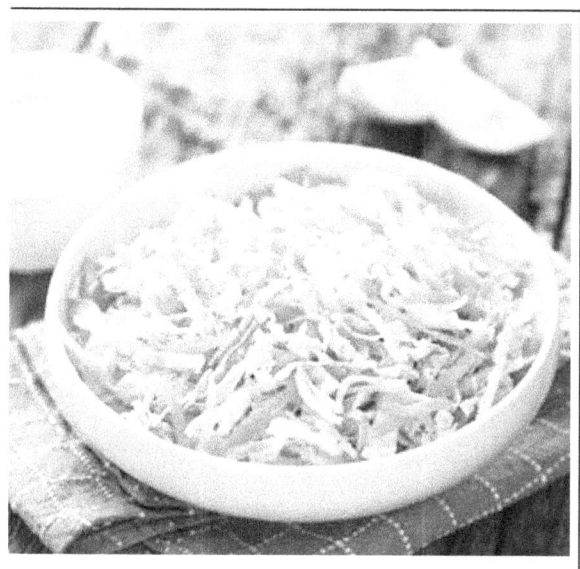

INGREDIENTS

- Shredded cabbage 1 and 1/2 cup.
- Grated carrots 2
- Bell pepper thinly sliced 1
- Cherry tomatoes 2 sliced.
- Green apple grated 1/2 cup.
- Sugar 1 teaspoon.
- Salt 1/4 teaspoon.
- Mayonnaise 1/4 cup.

Azerbaijan

Baku, Azerbaijan, is the capital of Azerbaijan. It has over 2 million populations.
The city is home to several impressive landmarks, including the Maiden Tower, the Blue Mosque, and the Baku Zoo.
Food and drinks in Azerbaijan include Shah Plov, Saj Ichi, Gutabs, Black tea, Ayran (yogurt mixed drink).
The Candy Cane Mountains, Flame Towers (the tallest skyscrapers), characterized by a wide variety of landscapes, skiing, and grand prix are considered as the best part of a trip to Azerbaijan.

DIRECTIONS

- Mix all vegetables.
- Add mayo, salt pepper, and mix well.

Georgia: Georgian Salad

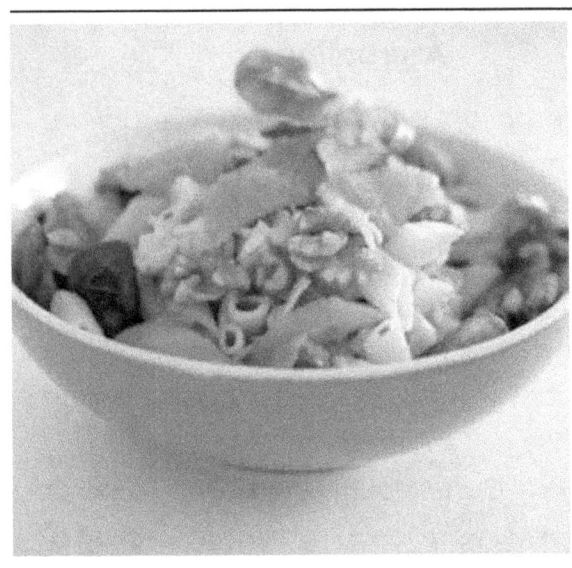

Georgia

Georgia has a unique history of ancient architecture, beautiful mountain and black seas. Its capital is Tbilisi.

Georgia is at the intersection of Europe and Asia, known as the original producer and birthplace of wine.

Fun things for tourists to do are biking, nature sights, hiking, bird shows, and caving.

INGREDIENTS

- Tomatoes 3 sliced
- Cucumber 2 sliced.
- Cilantro 1/4 cup chopped.
- Green chili for garnishing salad.
- Walnut dressing
- Walnut 2 tabspoon
- Vinegar 2 tabspoon.
- Garlic 1 chopped.
- Salt 1 pinch
- Black Pepper 1/4 teaspoon.

DIRECTIONS

- Add tomatoes, cucumbers, and cilantro in a bowl.
- Make a fine powder of walnuts in a pastel mirror or blender
- Whisk together vinegar, garlic, salt, and Pepper.
- Pour dressing over salad and enjoy.

Kyrgyz Republic: Special Salad

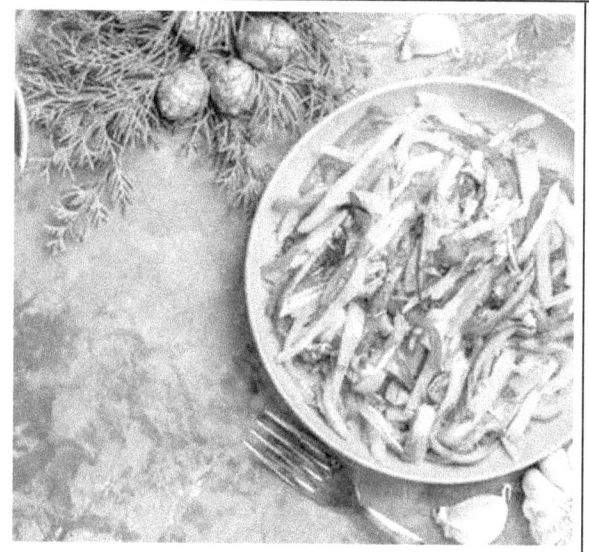

Kyrgyz Republic

*Kyrgyz Republic is a country in Central Asia. It is bordered by Kazakhstan Tajikistan, Uzbekistan, and China.
The capital and largest city is Bishkek. Walnut forests are famous all around the nation, traditional foods include lots of tea, horse meat and milk.
Kyrgyzstan is hilly and it is frequently called the "Switzerland" of Central Asia.*

INGREDIENTS

- Tomatoes 2 diced.
- Bell pepper 1 thinly sliced.
- Cucumber cut with peels 1
- Scallions 1 bunch chopped.
- Olive oil 2-tab spoon
- Lemon juice 2-tab spoon

DIRECTIONS

- Mix lemon juice, olive oil, some chopped scallion, salt, and black Pepper to form a dressing.
- Toss dressing with salad veggies and serve.

Nauru: Nauru Salad

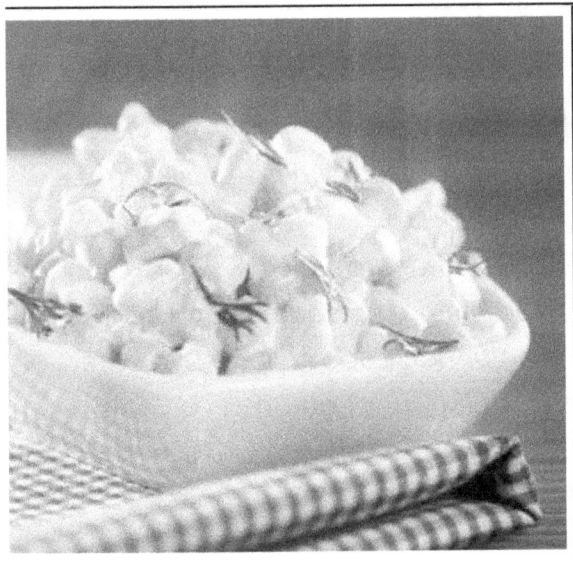

Nauru

Nauru was created in early 2001 as a resettlement site for people displaced by the East Timor genocide.

The site is in the outer reef of Nauru, approximately 1 kilometer north of the island's capital, Nauru.

The resettlement site initially accommodated 116 people but has grown to house over 1,400 people, including many refugees who have fled violence and persecution in the Middle East, Africa, and elsewhere.

INGREDIENTS

- Whole kernel corn, 1 can drained
- Tomato, 1 chopped
- Cucumber 1 chopped.
- Green pepper 1 chopped
- Green onion 1 chopped.
- Celery 1/4 cup chopped.
- Sour cream 1/4 cup
- Mayonnaise 2 tabspoon.
- Vinegar 1 tabspoon.
- Salt 1/4 teaspoon
- Crushed black pepper 1/4 teaspoon.

DIRECTIONS

- Mix sour cream, mayonnaise, vinegar, salt, and black pepper in a bowl.
- Add all vegetables plus dressing and toss well.
- Garnish with fresh parsley.

The Democratic Republic of the Congo: Congo Salad

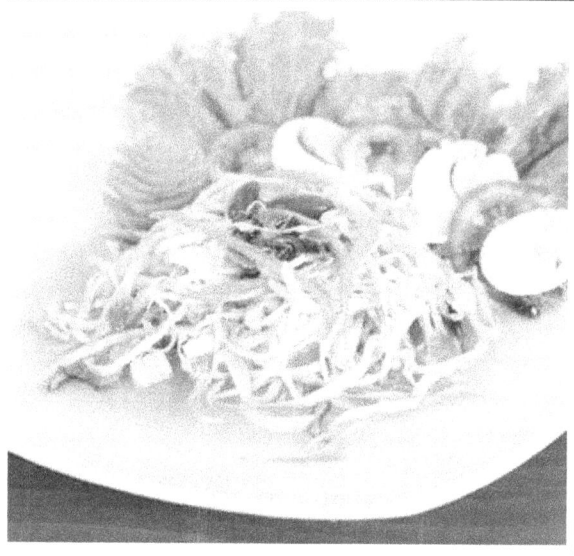

INGREDIENTS

- Cabbage shredded 1 and 1/2 cup
- Corn 1 cup use can corn for best results
- Hard-boiled eggs 3 cut into halves.
- Salad cream 4 tab spoon
- Salt 1/4 teaspoon
- Black Pepper 1/4 teaspoon

The Democratic Republic of the Congo

The Democratic Republic of the Congo is in Central Africa.
It is bordered by the Central African Republic, Rwanda, Uganda to the south, and Zambia.
The Congo is the second-largest country in Africa, with a population of over 58 million people.
The country is divided into six provinces. The capital of the Congo is Kinshasa.
The country's official languages are French and Lingala.

DIRECTIONS

- Mix all ingredients and refrigerate for 1/2 hour for best results.

Eritrea: Eritrean Salad

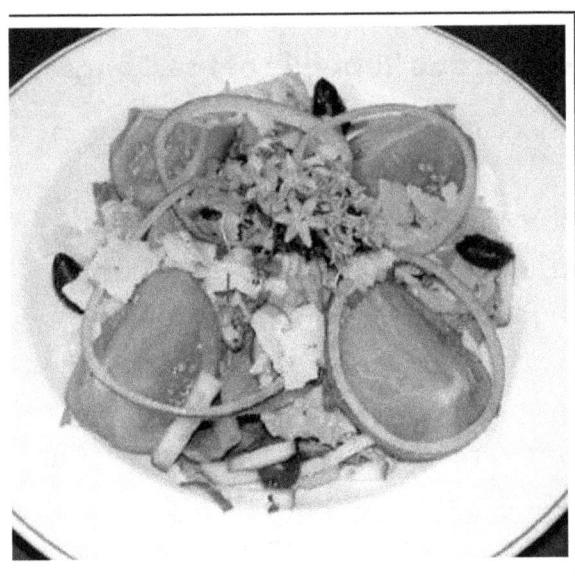

Eritrea

Eritrea is on the red seacoast and borders Sudan, Djibouti and Ethiopia.
Its capital is Asmara.
Eritrea has beautiful architecture buildings with influences from the Italians, Egyptians and Turkish.

INGREDIENTS

- Tomatoes 5 diced
- Red onions 2
- Garlic cloves
- Tomato paste 1-tab spoon.
- Jalapeno 1 diced.
- Crusty rolls toreinto pieces 4 ounces
- Cayenne Pepper
- All spice powder ¼ teaspoon.
- Salt 1/4 teaspoon.

DIRECTIONS

- Heat oil in a pan. Add half red onions and garlic. Cook until onions become soft and transparent.
- Add diced tomatoes, salt, paprika, cayenne, pepper, jalapeno, all spice powder, water, and ¼ cup in a bowl.
- Cook until tomatoes become tender. The sauce is ready.
- Presentation.
- Place bread into a serving bowl.
- Pour prepared tomato sauce,top with jalapeno
- Serve with Greek yogurt

Lesotho: Lesotho salad

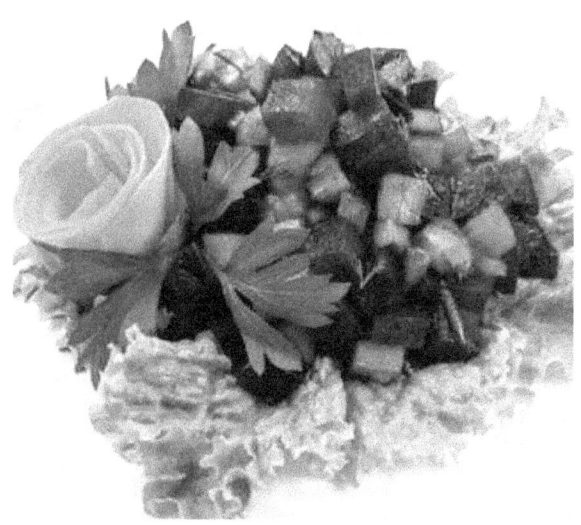

Lesotho

Lesotho is a small, landlocked country in southern Africa.
South Africa borders Lesotho Botswana, Congo as well.
Lesotho has a diverse culture with a strong traditional heritage.
The country is also home to several important natural resources, including mineral deposits and water resources.

INGREDIENTS

- Beets boiled and sliced 3
- Red onions 1 chopped
- Carrot 1 grated
- Olive oil 1 tabspoon.
- Apple cider vinegar 1 tabspoon

DIRECTIONS

- Satay onions and carrots for 1 minute on medium flame.
- Add grated beets and mix.
- Add apple cider vinegar. Mix well for 1 minute.

Gabon: Cucumber salad

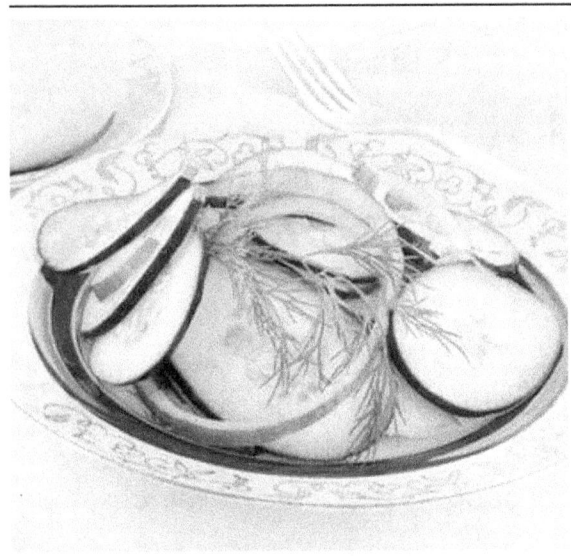

INGREDIENTS

- Cucumber 3 sliced
- Tomatoes 2 sliced
- Onions 1 thinly sliced.
- Fresh parsley 1/2 cup
- Fresh mint chopped 2 tabspoon.
- Salt ¼ teaspoon
- Crushed black Pepper ¼ teaspoon.
- Roasted cumin 1/2 teaspoon
- Olive oil 2 tabspoon.
- Lemon juice 1 tabspoon

Gabon

Gabon is in West Africa. It has a population of about 1.3 million people. Equatorial Guinea borders the country to the north, the Republic of the Congo to the east, and Congo to the south. Gabon is amazingly lovely and can possibly be one of the world's top points for ecotourism. Libreville is the capital city of Gabon.

Popular dishes are generally grilled/barbecued meat or fish and The local beer is Régab

Gabon is full of natural life, including swamp gorillas and chimpanzees, while imperiled turtles and whales on the Atlantic coast are fun for the tourists.

The country has a diverse culture, with a mixture of African, French, and Portuguese influences.

DIRECTIONS

- Mix tomatoes, onions, cucumbers, parsley, and fresh mint in a bowl.
- Add salt, black Pepper, olive oil, and lemon juice. Give it a gentle mix and serve.

Liberia: Potato salad

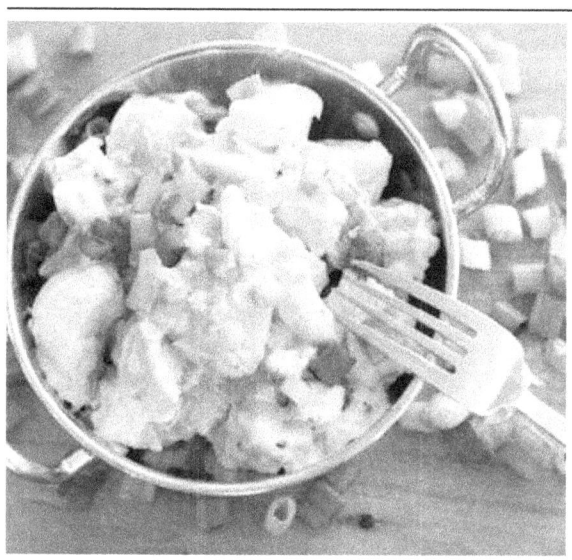

INGREDIENTS

- Russet potatoes 6 boiled and cubes
- Hard-boiled eggs 3 cut into half
- Green onion 2 tab spoon
- Mix veggies can 1 cup
- Dressing
- Mayonnaise ½ cup
- Cream ½ cup
- Garlic Salt 1 teaspoon.
- Black Pepper 1/4teaspoon.

Liberia

Liberia officially the Republic of Liberia, is on the West African seacoast.
Ivory Coast Frames Sierra Leone to its east, northwest, Guinea to its north, and the Atlantic Ocean to its south and southwest.
The cuisine is a mixed of meat, fish, vegetables, and spices and their ginger beer is considered as popular drink.
The Liberian National Museum, a coastal town with excellent surfing opportunities, and Omega Tower in Paynesville, known as the tallest structure in Africa
English is official language along with 20 indigenous languages, reflecting the country's ethnical and artistic diversity.
The country's capital and largest megacity is Monrovia

DIRECTIONS

- Add hard-boiled eggs, Mashed potatoes, mix veggies and green onions in a bowl.
- Mix cream, mayo, Pepper, garlic salt, and stir in salad veggies.
- Chill for ½ hour and then serve.

Ontario, Canada: Ontario Salad

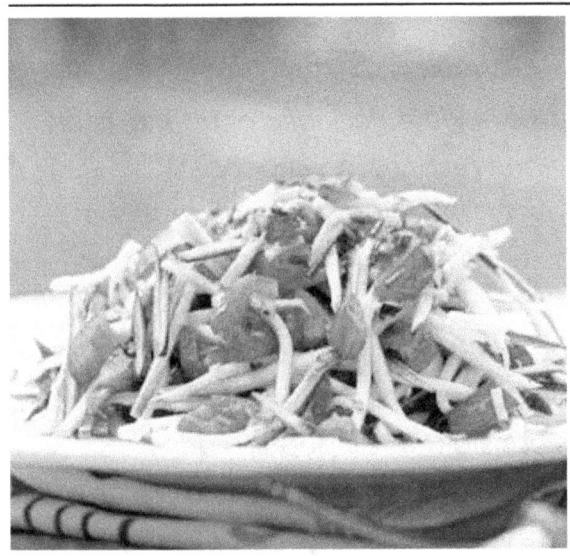

Ontario, Canada

Ontario province is situated in central Canada.
Ontario is the second-largest province in Canada, second only to Quebec.
Ontario is famous for its Cheddar cheese, maple syrup, pasta, shawarma, Caesar cocktail. a diverse array of cultures and languages.
Ontario's amazing charm is its freshwater lake, streams, and shore. Guests appreciate skating, skiing, and snowshoeing
Ontario is known for its natural resources and is a leading producer of agricultural products, energy, and steel.
Encounter amazing sights, sounds, flavors while embracing the metropolitan city.

INGREDIENTS

- Lettuce leaves 3-4
- Zucchini 1 thinly sliced
- Tomato 1 thinly sliced
- Carrot 1 thinly sliced
- Green beans 1 cup
- Green onion 1 chopped
- Vinegar 3 tab spoon.
- Olive oil 2 tab spoon
- Basil ½ tea spoon
- Salt ¼ teaspoon
- Black Pepper ¼ teaspoon.

DIRECTIONS

- Place tomatoes in a shallow dish.
- Set zucchini, carrots, tomato, green beans
- Shake dressing ingredients well
- Pour dressing on the salad.
- Chill for 1-hour l before serving.

San Carlos, Mexico: Cabbage Salad

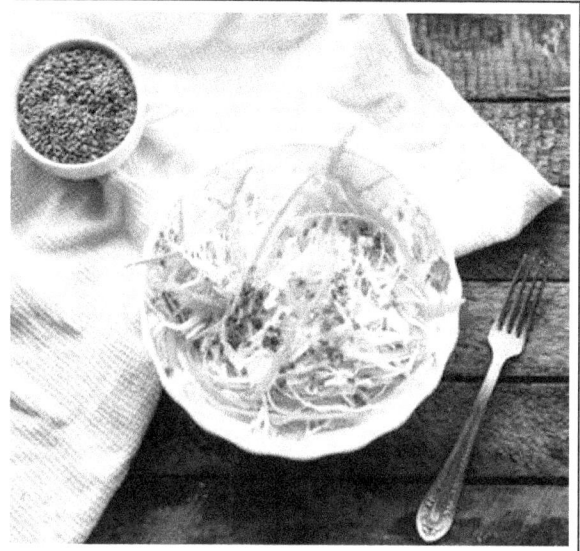

INGREDIENTS

- Cabbage shredded 1 cup
- Carrot 1 thinly sliced.
- Fresh cilantro chopped 1/2 cup
- Olive oil 2 tab spoon
- Rice Vinegar 4 tab spoon
- Salt ¼ teaspoon
- Crushed Black Pepper 1/4 teaspoon.

San Carlos, Mexico

San Carlos is a small town located in the state of Michoacán, Mexico.
This delightful city, the capital of Cojedes Estado, is surrounded by desert, low-lying mountains, marinas and the beaches. Cocktails, grilled meat and wines keep tourists refreshed throughout their travel. In the summer try the water sports and fishing and winter hiking, climbing, biking, horseback riding, and sightseeing.
San Carlos known for its hand-woven textile, pottery and warm hospitality.

DIRECTIONS

- Mix oil, vinegar, salt, Pepper, and fresh cilantro
- Stir in carrots, cabbage and toss well

Puerto Vallarta, Mexico: Puerto Vallarta salad

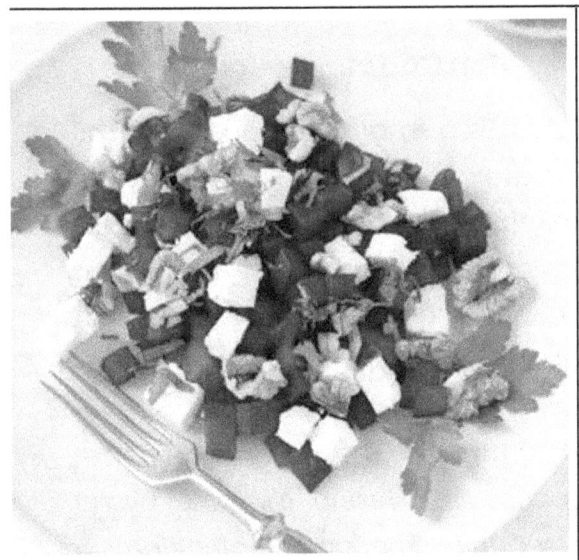

Puerto Vallarta, Mexico

Puerto Vallarta is a beautiful city on Mexico's Pacific Coast

It is known for its clear blue waters and white sand beaches. The city is also home to many restaurants and shops.

Puerto Vallarta is a great place to relax and enjoy the beautiful beaches and scenery.

INGREDIENTS

- Beets boiled 3
- Arugula 2 leaves.
- Fresh broccoli 1 cup
- Fried Brussels sprouts 1 cup.
- Feta cheese or Mac and cheese
- Olive oil 2 tab spoon
- Apple cider vinegar 2 tab spoon.
- Lime juice of 1 lime.
- Sugar 1 pinch.

DIRECTIONS

- Mix all vegetables, and season with salt, Pepper.
- Squeeze lime juice, and here you go!

Miami, Florida: Miami salad

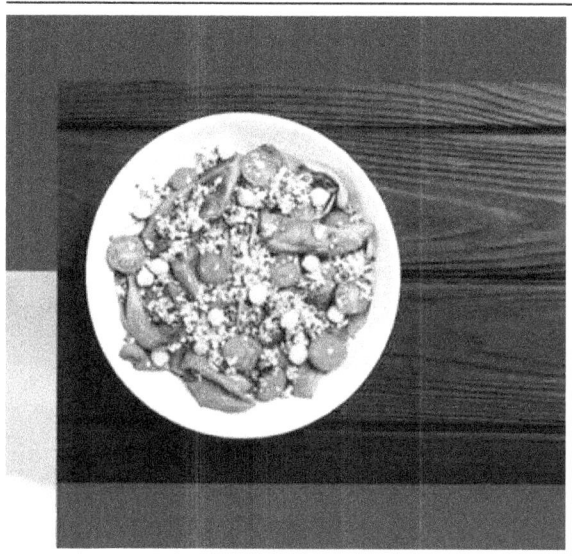

INGREDIENTS

- Baby Romaine lettuce 2 cups.
- Sweet potatoes boiled and cubed 1 cup.
- Corn 1 cup.
- Baby spinach 1 cup
- Scallion 2
- Artichoke hearts
- Green bell pepper 1 thinly sliced.
- Avocados 3 sliced.
- Black olives 10 sliced
- Dill pickle 2
- White wine vinegar 2 tabspoon
- Olive oil 1/2 cup
- Garlic cloves 2 chopped.
- Dijon mustard 1/2 teaspoon.
- Honey 1/4 teaspoon.
- Salt 1 pinch
- Pepper 1/4 teaspoon

Miami, Florida

Miami, Florida, also known as "The Magic City" of Florida, is the most popular vacation spot because of its night life, beaches, fun-filled entertainment and shopping.
Cuban sandwiches, Cuban bread, pork, and cheese are popular foods in Miami.
Their traditional drinks include mojitos, strawberry & milkshakes,
The city is home to the Coconut Grove Festival, lots of entertainment places, museums, theaters.
Next time you are in Miami try Jungle Island, Bayfront Park, & Miami Zoo.

DIRECTIONS

- Mix dressing ingredients well.
- Add all vegetables into the serving bowl.
- Pour dressing onto the salad.
- Serve immediately.

Portland, Oregon: Portland salad

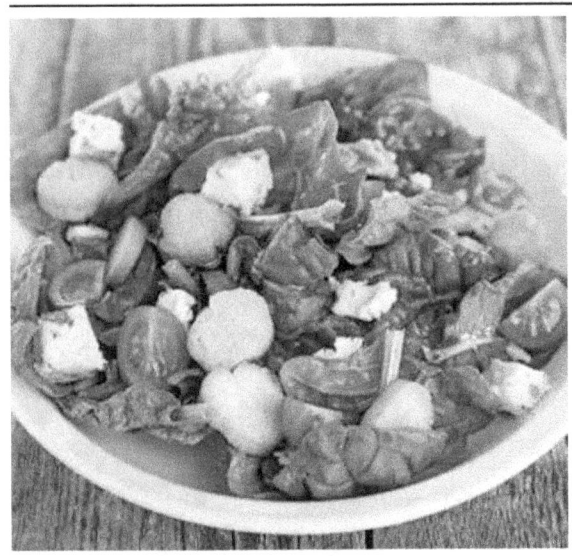

Portland, Oregon

Portland is a city of the United States Oregon. The city is famous for its stunning waterfront, lively nightlife, and many parks.
There are also several interesting museums and cultural sites to visit.
Portland is a great place to play, work and live.
Next time you visit check out their pizza, coffee, wine, street food and cocktails during your trip.

INGREDIENTS

- Spinach 1 cup
- Shredded cabbage 1 and 1/2 cup.
- Arugula 2 -3 leaves
- Avocado 1 sliced
- Cucumber 2 sliced
- Pickled onions 1 chopped
- Carrots 1 thinly sliced.
- Salt Black Pepper
- Ranch dressing 1/4 cup.

DIRECTIONS

- Mix all ingredients and enjoy your meal.

Greece: Greek salad

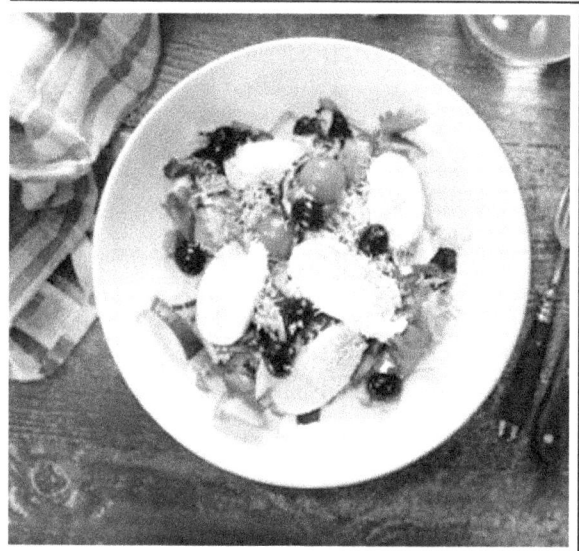

INGREDIENTS

- Green pepper 1 chopped
- Grape tomatoes 1 cup
- Cucumber sliced 1
- Red onion 1 chopped
- Vinegar 2-tab spoon.
- Olive oil 1-tab spoon.
- Greek oregano 1 teaspoon
- Kalamata olives 10
- Feta cheese crumbled 1/4 cup.
- 1 teaspoon dried basil

Greece

Greece is in southeastern Europe. It has a long and complex history. The first inhabitants of Greece were the Minoans, who lived on the island of Crete from the Late Neolithic period until the Bronze Age.

The beautiul mountains and beaches draw sightseers from a long way off.

Lemons and tomatoes are must haves in their food and olive oil is a staple in Greek cooking.

Bread and wine are constantly served during supper, as well as pork, chicken, and other meats.

The most-visited places in Greece are Mykonos, Olympia, Rhodes, and Crete and the Panoramic view of Oia will blow your mind away.

DIRECTIONS

- Add all veggies in a bowl.
- Add olive oil and vinegar.
- Top with feta cheese and olives.

Croatia: Croatian salad

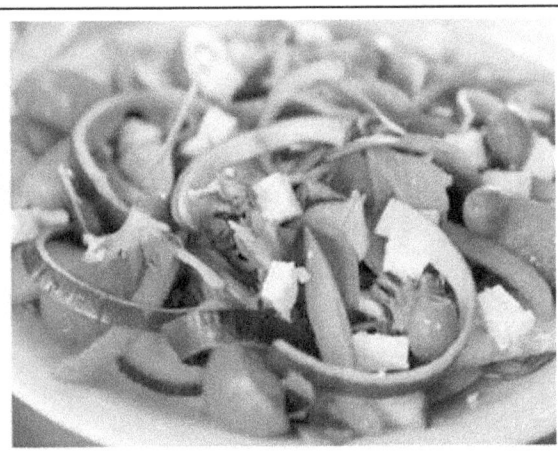

Croatia

Croatia is a Balkan country located in Southeast Europe.
Slovenia borders it to the west, Hungary, Serbia to the north, Bosnia and Herzegovina, Montenegro, Macedonia to the east, and Italy to the south with
Low mountains and highlands close to the Adriatic coastline.
Winters are cold and blanketed summers are gentle.
The capital and largest city is Zagreb. Popular food are tendered meat and vegetable dish Peka
traditional Rakija (herbal drink).
The co Plitvička Lakes National Park, Hvar, the Cathedral of Zagreb, and Diocletian's Palace are the best
known places to visit in this country.

INGREDIENTS

- Onion 1 round slices
- Cucumber 2 thinly sliced
- Tomatoes 2 diced
- Red pepper 2 chopped.
- Olive oil 2-tab spoon
- Vinegar 2-tab spoon
- Salt 1 pinch
- Black Pepper

DIRECTIONS

- Mix all veggies, sprinkle salt, Pepper, add lemon juice, and toss well.

Albania: Albanian salad

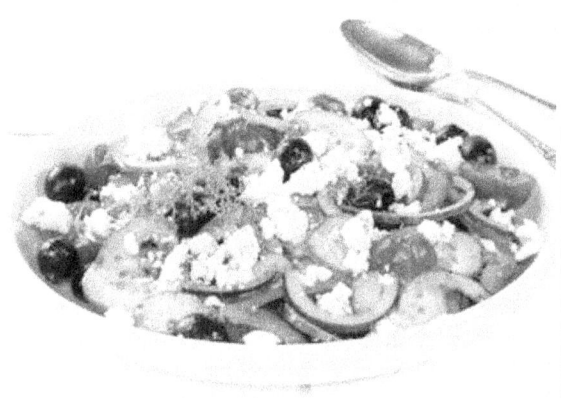

Albania

Albania is a small, landlocked country in the heart of Europe.
It is made up of a mountainous interior and a Mediterranean coastline.
The capital and largest city is Tiran.
It has over 3 million populations. Albanians are generally hospitable people and enjoy a high standard of living.
They are proud of their traditional history and enjoy rich folklore.

INGREDIENTS

- Tomatoes 2 sliced
- Cucumber 1 sliced
- Green bell pepper 1 thinly sliced.
- Black olives 10 sliced
- Salt 1/4 teaspoon.
- Crushed Black Pepper 1/4 teaspoon.
- Feta cheese crumble 1/4 cup.

DIRECTIONS

- Mix all ingredients together and simply enjoy!

Lithuania: Lithuanian white salad.

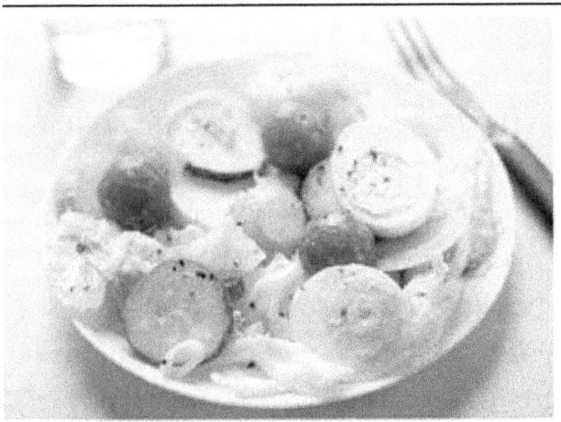

Lithuania

Lithuania is a small country of Baltic region. It has a population of just over 2 million, making it one of the least populous countries in Europe.

Lithuania is also one of the most sparsely populated countries in the world.

This makes it a very rural country, with only about 25% of the population living in urban areas.

Lithuania is ethnically and linguistically diverse, with a population that includes people from a wide range of European and Asian cultures.

Tourists enjoy their baked pastries, potato pancakes, pickles, and soup and the reviving non-alcoholic cocktail produced using rye bread drink.

INGREDIENTS

- Potatoes boiled and cubed 2
- Pickled Cucumber 3
- Carrots 2 thinly sliced.
- Canned peas 1/2 cup.
- Hard-boiled eggs 3 cut into cubes.
- Salt 1/4 teaspoon.
- Crushed Black Pepper 1/4 teaspoon.
- Mayonnaise 6 tab spoon.

DIRECTIONS

- Mix all vegetables. Sprinkle salt, crushed Black Pepper, mayonnaise, and toss well.
- Serve immediately

North Macedonia: North Macedonian salad

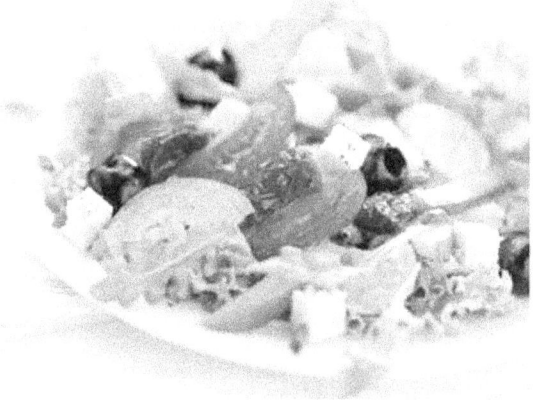

North Macedonia

It is a landlocked country which is in the Balkan Peninsula.
Serbia borders it to the northwest, Bulgaria to the northeast, Greece to the east, and Albania to the south.
The capital and largest city is Skopje. Pizza, baked beans, and stuffed rolls are perfect to amaze your tastebuds. Turkish coffee and Rakija are famous liquors of this country.

INGREDIENTS

- Onion 1 sliced.
- Cucumber 2 sliced.
- Tomato 3 sliced
- Green bell pepper 1 thinly sliced.
- Feta cheese crumble 1/4 cup.
- Fresh parsley 2 tab spoon.
- Salt 1 pinch
- Crushed Black Pepper 1/4 teaspoon.

DIRECTIONS

- Mix all veggies, season with salt, black Pepper,

Section 111

Pasta Salads

If you love pasta? and want to explore new exciting pasta recipes? Then you'll love for sure our PASTA SALAD RECIPES across the globe. This dish is flavorful and can be served as a light lunch or dinner. In addition to being delicious, this salad is also packed with nutrients, including vitamin A, vitamin C, and potassium.

There are many delicious ways to cook pasta salads. Here are a few tips:

- *Choose a variety of pasta shapes and colors.*
- *Mix together a variety of salad ingredients.*
- *Drizzle your pasta salad with a delicious dressing.*

El Salvador: El Salvadorian salad

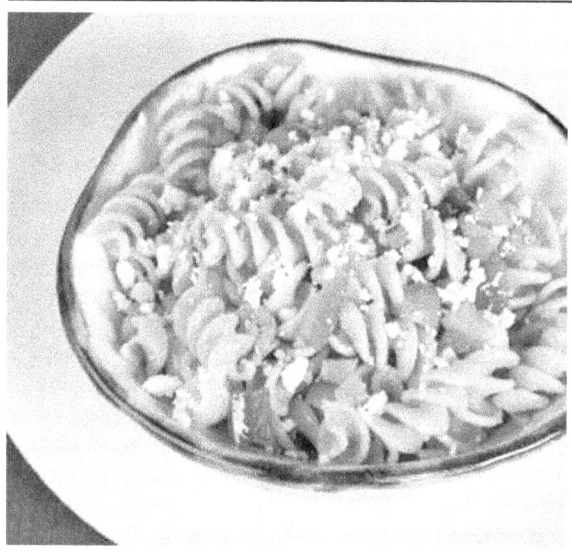

INGREDIENTS

- Pasta boiled 1 cup.
- Cabbage shredded 1 and 1/2 cup.
- Carrot 1 thinly sliced.
- Green onion 2 chopped.
- Hot water 1 cup
- Vinegar 1 cup
- Water 1/2 cup
- Oregano 1 tabspoon.
- Salt 1/4 teaspoon
- Black Pepper 1/4 teaspoon

El Salvador

El Salvador is in Central America and has a population of approximately six million people, mostly of indigenous and mixed races.

Honduras borders the country to the north, Guatemala to the south, and the Pacific Ocean to the east.

It is known for its volcanoes and it is the only country that does not have a coastline on the Caribbean Sea.

Rice, beans, and tortillas are popular dishes. Their traditional drink is Atole de elote a mixture of sugar, cinnamon, and corn.

DIRECTIONS

- Boil cabbage and carrots in boiling water for 5 minutes.
- Drain and cool veggies.
- Then add green onions, pasta, vinegar, water, salt, black pepper, dried oregano, and toss well.

French Guiana: French Guiana salad

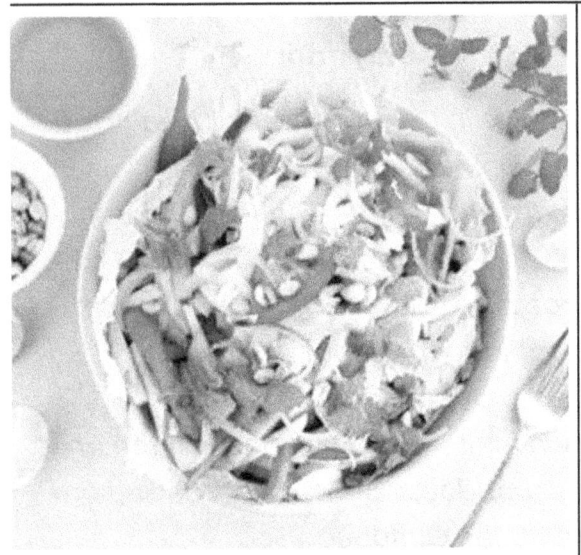

INGREDIENTS

- Pasta boiled 1 cup.
- Green mangoes 2 small sized.
- Onion chopped 1/4 cup.
- Garlic cloves peeled and chopped 2
- Chili pepper chopped 1/2 or paprika powder 1/4 teaspoon.
- Olive oil 2 tab spoon
- Lemon juice 2 tab spoon
- Salt 1/4 teaspoon
- Crushed black pepper 1/4 teaspoon.
- Shrimps cooked 12
- Instructions.
- Peel green mangoes and shred the pulp.
- Add salt, black pepper, lemon juice, onions, mix, and chill for 2 hours.

French Guiana

French Guiana is located on the north coast of the South American continent, bordered by Suriname Brazil and the Atlantic Ocean. French Guiana was originally inhabited by indigenous people, most of the country is rainforest with beautiful creoles houses and colorful street markets.

The food is exceptionally assorted Bouillon d'Awara, lentils, and Colombo are popular. The local rum of this nation is the best reviving beverage for travelers.

The seaside fields rising to hills and small mountains are a speculator experience.

DIRECTIONS

- Pour salad onto the serving platter .Set pasta.
- Place shrimps around green mango mixture.
- Garnish with parsley.

Paraguay: Paraguay salad

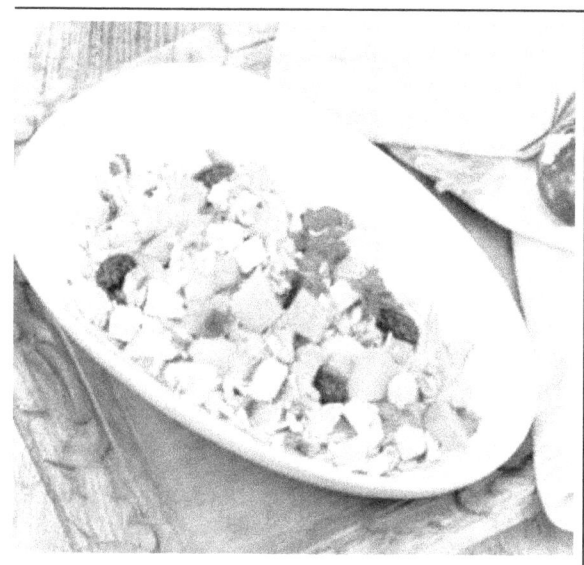

Paraguay

Paraguay is in the South American continent with a population of just over 6 million people. Brazil, Bolivia and Argentina borders it.

The climate is humid and warm, Paraguay is rich in natural resources, including gold, silver, iron, copper, etc.

Paraguayan Soup, Corn Cake, Cheddar and Starch Bread, Cheddar Flatbread, and patties are popular dishes, along by the national beverage Yerba Mate.

INGREDIENTS

- Pasta boiled 1 cup.
- Cassava peeled and cut into slices 2 cups.
- Pumpkin peeled and cut into chunks 2 cups.
- Onion 1 chopped
- Garlic 2 cloves minced.
- Eggs hard-boiled 2 cut into halves.
- Mayonnaise 1 cup
- Salt 1/4 teaspoon
- Crushed Black pepper 1/4 teaspoon.

DIRECTIONS

- Mix mayonnaise, salt, black pepper, vinegar, and sugar in a bowl.
- Add dressing to all veggies and toss well.

The Bahamas: Bahamian pasta salad

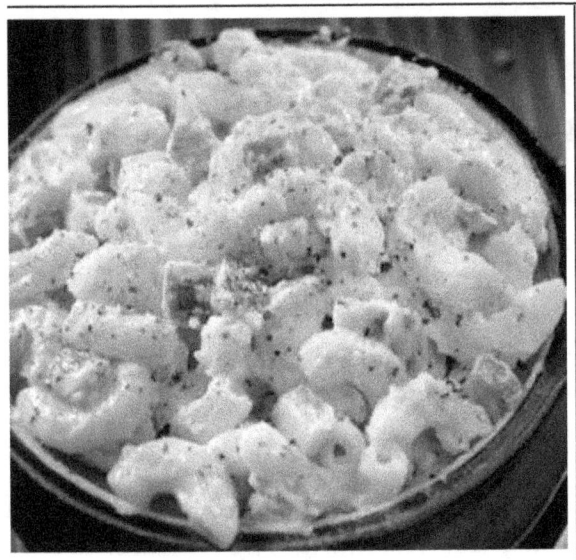

INGREDIENTS

- Boiled pasta 1 cup
- Lemon zest 1 tabspoon
- Fresh dill 1/2 cup chopped.
- Salmon Cooked 1 fillet or shrimp cooked 1 cup
- Parmesan cheese 2 tabspoon
- Heavy cream 1 cup.
- Salt 1/4 teaspoon
- Black Pepper 1/4 teaspoon
- Asparagus boiled 1/2 cup

The Bahamas

The Bahamas is a small island in the middle of the Atlantic Ocean. The islands are beautiful, with crystal-clear water and white sand beaches.

The climate is tropical, and the islands are known for their crystal-clear water and white sand beaches. The people are hospitable, and there are a lot of activities to enjoy, including diving, snorkeling, sailing, and windsurfing.

The Bahamas is a great place to relax and escape city life.

DIRECTIONS

- Add heavy cream, dill, lemon zest, and parmesan cheese in a pan and cook until the sauce thickens.
- Stir in pasta and asparagus
- Top with prepared salmon and some fresh parsley

Guyana: Guyanese pasta salad.

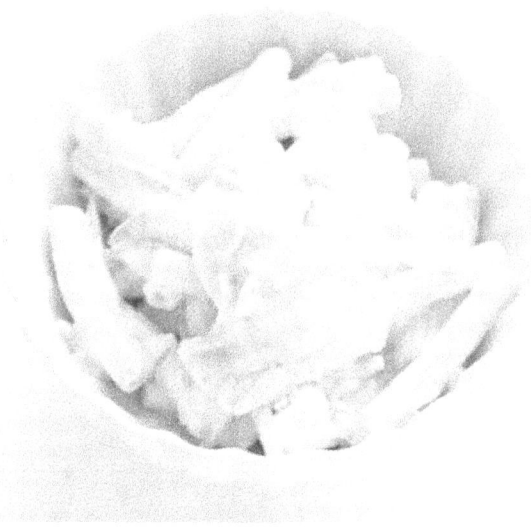

Guyana

The Land of many waters and Oil Rich Guyana are phases use to describe Guyana. The capital city of is Georgetown. Guyana is a very diverse country with a mix of cultures. They are African, Indian, Chinese, Portuguese, Mixed, and Amerindian.

The main crops in the country are rice, sugarcane, bauxite, gold and diamonds. Bake and salt fish, barbecued fish, and cooked-up rice are their must-have food As well as the sorrel, mauby, cane juice and fruit punch.

INGREDIENTS

- Pasta
- Elbow macaroni boiled 1 cup
- Tie bow pasta ¼ cup
- Garlic butter 1 tabspoon.
- Mustard 1tabspoon
- Mayonnaise 1 cup
- Spicy mayonnaise or peri sauce 1 tabspoon.
- Hot sauce 1 tabspoon.
- Cream 1/4 cup
- Evaporated milk 1/4 cup
- Cottage cheese 2 tabspoon
- Carrot 1 thinly sliced.
- Spring onions 1 chopped.
- Wine or rum 1/2 teaspoon.
- Salt 1/4 teaspoon.
- Crushed Black pepper 1/4 teaspoon.

DIRECTIONS

- Add veggies, mayonnaise, milk, cream, and cottage cheese to the bowl.
- Mix thoroughly

Barbados: Bajan salad

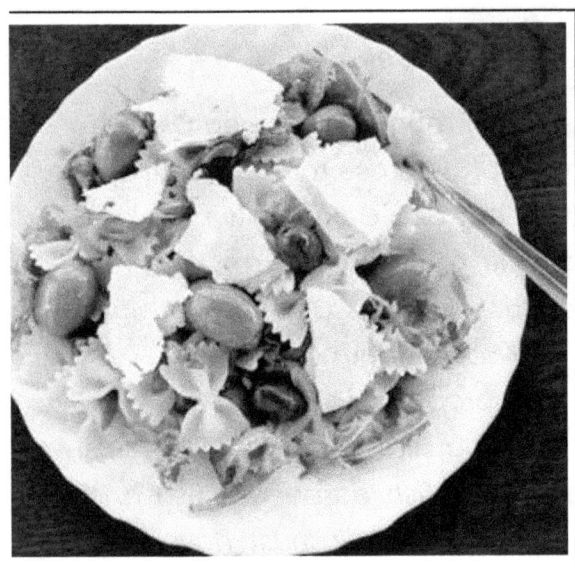

Barbados

Barbados is a tiny island country located in the eastern Caribbean Sea. The country is known for its beautiful beaches, lively nightlife, and lush rainforest.
The Coral island of Barbados offers you in excess of 80 perfect white-sand sea shores and delicious West Indian curries, roti, meat, and Caribbean food.

INGREDIENTS

- Elbow macaroni boiled 2 cups
- Red onion chopped 1
- Green bell pepper 1 chopped.
- Evaporated milk 1/2 cup.
- Ketchup 5 tabspoon
- Mustard 1 teaspoon.
- Honey 1 teaspoon.
- Salt 1/4 teaspoon
- Onion Powder 1/2 teaspoon
- Garlic powder 1/4 teaspoon.
- Crushed Black pepper 1/2 teaspoon.
- Thyme 1/2 teaspoon.
- Onion powder 1/2 teaspoon.
- Feta cheese grated 1/4 cup.

DIRECTIONS

- Mix all ingredients
- Top with feta cheese.
- Refrigerate for 1/2 hour and then serve

Saint Vincent and the Grenadines: Pasta Salad

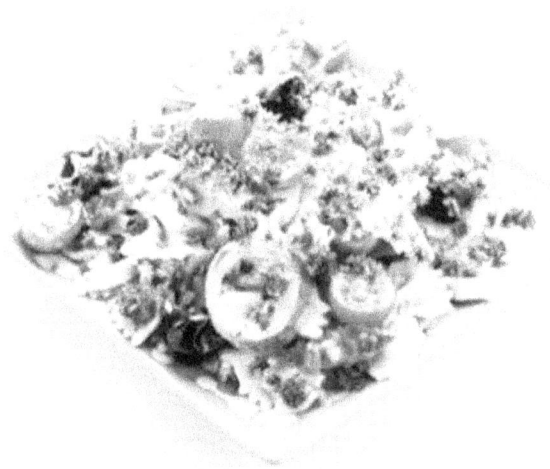

Saint Vincent and the Grenadines

St Vincent and the Grenadines, a multi-island nation. The islands are renowned for diving and calming beaches. The capital city is Kingstown. Callaloo soup, fish, banana squanders, and Hairoun Beer are their preferred foods and beverages. Delightful bayous and fine beaches represent rich vacationers. St. Vincent and the Grenadines procured the best position in the Caribbean and is additionally known for yachting and sailing.

INGREDIENTS

- Rotini pasta boiled 2 cups.
- Whole kernel corn 1 cup.
- Black beans 1 cup.
- Roma tomatoes chopped 1/2 cup.
- Red bell pepper chopped 1
- Green bell pepper chopped 1
- Olive oil 2 tabspoon
- Lime juice 2 tabspoon
- Fresh cilantro 1/4 cup.

DIRECTIONS

- Mix all vegetables and pasta.
- Add olive oil, lime juice and mix well.
- Serve chill for best results.

Grenada: Grenadian Pasta Salad

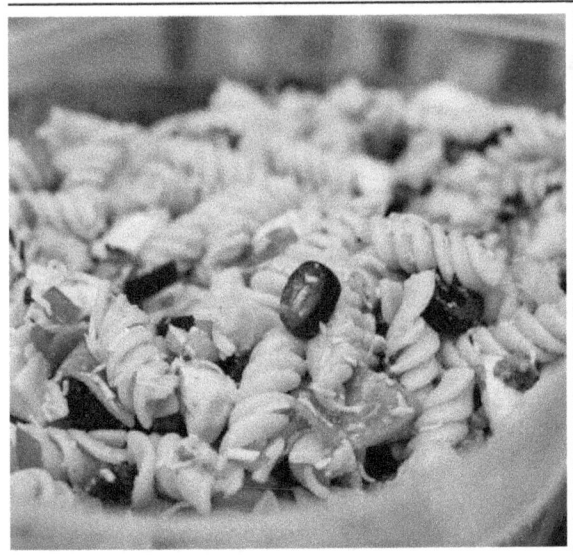

Grenada

A nation in the Caribbean, or West Indies and is known as the "Spice Isle", being a significant producer of cocoa, nutmeg, cloves, ginger, cinnamon, and vanilla. Their local fruit smoothie, rum, grilled meat, cheese burgers, and sushi are truly enjoyed by tourists.
Morne Rouge Ocean side, Annandale waterfalls, and Market in St. George's are must visits for explorers. The island is a popular diving destination, with many dive sites accessible by boat.

INGREDIENTS

- Farfalle pasta boiled 2 cups
- Sun-dried tomatoes 2 cups
- Pine nuts 1/4 cup
- Parmesan cheese grated 1/4 cup
- Feta cheese crumbled 1/4 cup.
- Fresh dill 2-tab spoon
- Parsley 2-tab spoon
- Basil leaves 2-tab spoon.
- Olive oil 2-tab spoon
- Lime juice 2-tab spoon
- Crushed red chili 1/2 teaspoon
- Salt 1/4 teaspoon.

DIRECTIONS

- Blend sun-dried tomatoes, vinegar, oil, pine nuts, crushed red chili, Parmesan, salt, and crushed red pepper.
- Add this paste to boiled pasta.
- Mix well.
- Garnish with fresh parsley.

Tajikistan: Tajikistan Salad 'Qurtob'

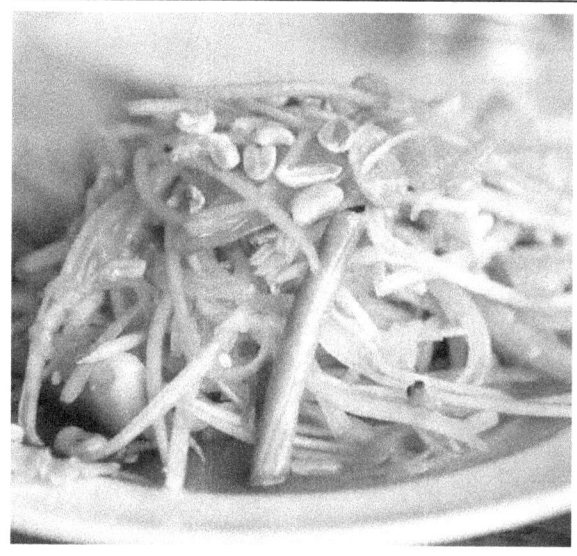

Tajikistan

Tajikistan in Central Asia, Tajikistan. The capital and biggest city of Tajikistan is Dushanbe.

Their national dish is plov (rice with meat or chicken), and the national drink is green tea. There are many things to explore in Tajikistan. The country is rich in natural resources, including agricultural land, mineral deposits, and water reserves.

INGREDIENTS

- 1 cup (80 g) Greek yogurt
- 200 ml fresh cream
- 1 cucumber
- 1 tomato
- 1 small onion
- Green onion
- bread
- 50 g butter
- salt

DIRECTIONS

- Chop Vegetables cucumber, green tomato, green onion & onion.
- Add Greek yogurt, cream & butter,
- Mix well.
- Spread on bread.

Uzbekistan: Lagman Uzbek Noodle Salad

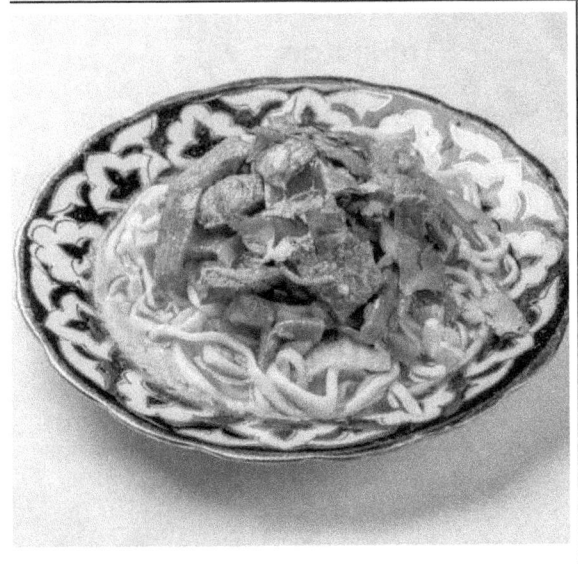

Uzbekistan

Uzbekistan is in Central Asia Tashken is the capital and biggest city.
Mouth-watering dishes of Tajikistan include meat skewers, soup, plov, and samsa. And their best beverages are green tea and vodka.
It is renowned for its traditional craftsmanship, including textiles, ceramics, and metalwork.

INGREDIENTS

- 2 tablespoons olive oil
- 1 onion, finely chopped
- ½ pound beef chuck, cut into strips
- 1 teaspoon ground cumin
- ½ teaspoon ground black pepper
- 2 tablespoons tomato paste
- 1 carrot, cut into thin strips
- 1 green bell pepper, cut into 1-inch strips
- 3 small potatoes, cubed
- ½ cup thinly sliced celery
- 8 cups water
- 2 teaspoons salt
- ½ cup finely chopped parsley
- 3 large cloves garlic, minced
- 2 (8 ounce) packages thin Chinese noodles

DIRECTIONS

- Heat oil in a large pot over high heat. Reduce heat to medium-high; cook and stir onion in hot oil until golden, 3 to 5 minutes. Stir in beef strips, cumin, and black pepper; cook until beef is browned, about 5 minutes. Stir in tomato paste and cook for 2 to 3 minutes.
- Stir carrot into the pot; cook until coated with tomato paste, 2 to 3 minutes. Add green bell pepper; cook for 1 minute. Add potatoes and celery; cook for 5 minutes. Pour in water; bring to a boil. Season water with salt. Reduce heat to low and simmer soup until potatoes are soft, about 40 minutes.
- Stir parsley and garlic into the soup. Simmer until garlic is soft, 10 to 15 minutes.
- Bring a large pot of lightly salted water to a boil. Cook noodles in boiling water, stirring occasionally, until tender yet firm to the bite, 3 to 5 minutes. Rinse and drain well. Divide among serving bowls. Ladle hot soup over noodles.

Asia

Afghanistan: Afghan Pasta Salad

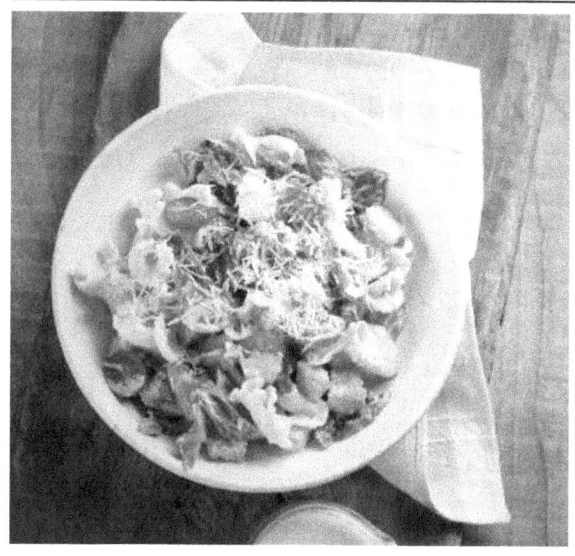

Afghanistan

Afghanistan, Kabul is the capital city. Popular dishes are Naan, Lavash, pulao, like Kabuli pulao, yakhni pulao, and Zamarod Pulao.

The green tea is popular beverage. Afghanistan is a blend of various societies, with Pashtuns, Tajiks, Hazaras, and Uzbeks comprising the biggest ethnic gatherings. Major exports are minerals, nuts, carpets, and wool.

INGREDIENTS

- 1 can tomato (s)
- 6 onion (s)
- 1 clove garlic
- 1 hot pepper, hot
- 1 tablespoon balsamic vinegar
- 1 tablespoon honey
- salt and pepper
- 250 g quark, (with 40% fat)
- a lot peppermint, dried
- 100 ml cream
- Tortellini

DIRECTIONS

- Cook the tortellini in a saucepan with salted water.
- Preparation of the red sauce:
- Sauté the onions and garlic in a pan with a little olive oil. Then add the chopped peppers. Then add the peeled tomatoes. Finally stir in honey and balsamic vinegar and season with salt and pepper.
- Preparation of the white sauce:
- Mix the quark and cream to a liquid sauce and add the dried peppermint.
- Put in the fridge and let it steep.
- Put the tortellini on a plate, then pour the red sauce over it and finally add a little more of the white sauce.
- Totally easy and quick! And super delicious! Just try!

Bangladesh: Bengali Pasta Salad

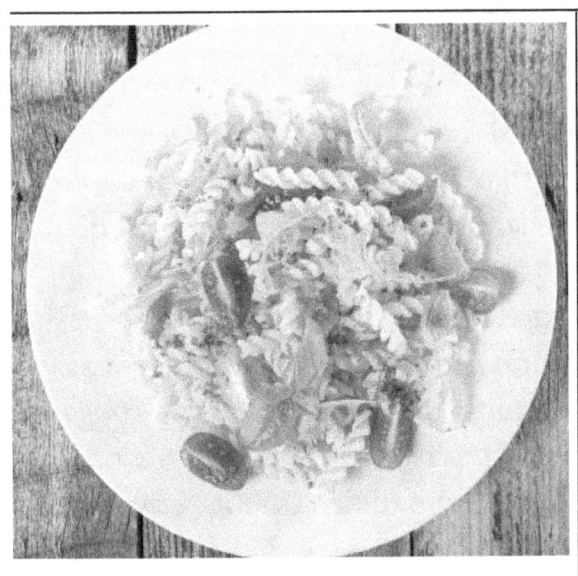

Bangladesh

Bangladesh is perhaps the most homogeneous country on the planet. Dhaka is the capital of Bangladesh.
The country has a diverse geography with forests, mountains, rivers, and delta regions. Dhaka fish and coconut oil in preparing dishes .
Coconut water and lassi are their traditional beverages.

INGREDIENTS

- 1 cup pasta
- Boiled mix vegetables (Peas, broccoli, carrots)
- 1 small chopped tomato
- 1 slice chopped onion
- 1 to 2 tbsp. Mayonnaise Cheese
- 50 gm of grated Mozzarella cheese
- few fresh springs of finely chopped Parsley
- 1 tsp. Seasonings
- 1/4 cup sliced stuffed olives
- 1 teaspoon soy sauce
- 1 tsp lemon juice
- Salt as per taste
- Black pepper powder

DIRECTIONS

- First you take the cooked pasta in widely deep bowl, blend all the ingredients such as boiled mixed vegetables, chopped onions and tomato in the bowl.
- Add the soy sauce, mayonnaise cheese, lemon juice and seasonings on top and mix well.
- Add black pepper and salt as per your taste.
- Sprinkle the chopped olives, finely chopped parsely and grated Mozzarella cheese on top of the salad.
- Keep in the refrigerator to make it chill for around 45 minutes.
- Once it get chilled lightly then mix again and see the taste.
- Pasta salad is ready to serve, you will simply love this recipe for sure.

Bhutan: Britain Pasta Salad

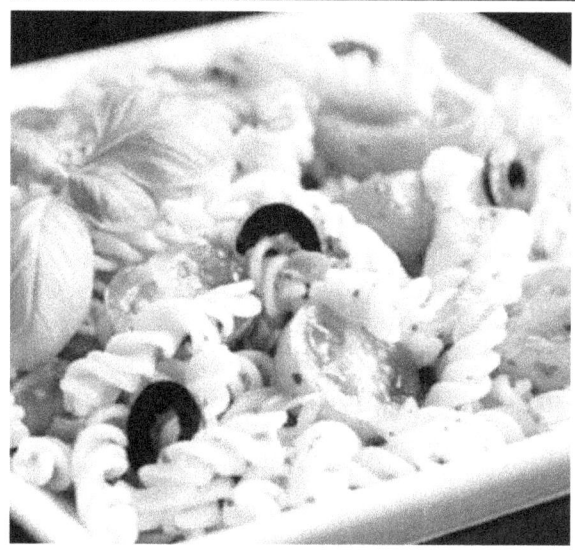

INGREDIENTS

- Cabbage shredded 2 cups.
- Red onion 1 chopped
- Peas 1 cup.
- Carrots 2 thinly sliced
- Roasted Almonds 1/4 cup
- Raisins 1/4 cup
- Pineapple cubes 1/4 cup
- Chicken breast 2 cut into cubes.
- For sauce.
- Ingredients
- Apple cider vinegar 4 tabspoon.
- Honey 5 tabspoon
- Sesame seeds 3 tabspoon.
- Soy sauce 2 tabspoon.
- Lemon juice 2 tabspoon.
- Crushed Black pepper 1/4 teaspoon.
- Salt 1/2 teaspoon.

Bhutan

Bhutan is a country in southern Asia between Tibet and India known for its stunning landscapes and Buddhist culture. Most of the population are ethnic Bhutanese, Buddhist monks, and nuns.
Ema dashti (chilli pepper and cheese soup), and Ara (alcoholic) are their national food and drink.
Bhutan is a great place to visit if you are looking for a peaceful environment and a place to learn about Buddhist culture.

DIRECTIONS

- First of all, for making sauce, mix honey, salt, apple cider vinegar, soy sauce, and lemon juice. Set aside.
- Heat 2 tabspoon oil, and add ginger garlic paste and chicken.Satay until 90% cook. Add prepared sauce to
- the cooked chicken and cook until the mixture thickens.
- Mix all veggies to this sauce-coated chicken and serve.

Fiji: Fiji Pasta Salad

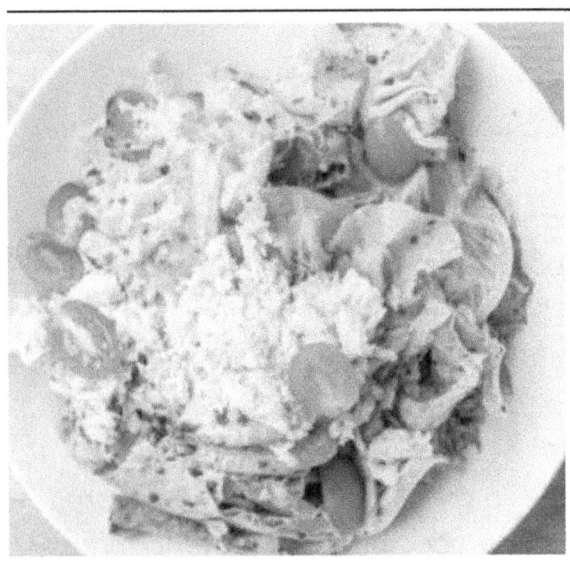

INGREDIENTS

- Pasta boiled 2 cups
- Tomatoes 2 chopped
- Onion 1 chopped
- Green chilies 1 chopped.
- Sweet chili sauce 1 tabspoon.
- Olive oil 1 tabspoon
- Butter 1 tabspoon.
- Lemon zest 1
- Lemon juice 2 tab spoon.
- Salt 1/2 teaspoon.
- Crushed black Pepper ¼ teaspoon.
- Canned tuna 1 drained
- Evaporated milk 1/2 cup

Fiji

The Republic of Fiji, is an archipelago of over 300 islands, with just over 100 inhabited It is located in the heart of the South Pacific, neighbors are Samoa, to the northeast, to the southwest Vanuatu, to the west, New Caledonia, to the southwest, Samoa, to the northeast, Tuvalu, to the north, and Tonga, to the east.

Fiji is known for its tropical fruits, such as pineapples, mangoes, and bananas. Popular foods in Fiji include kokoda, a raw fish dish marinated in coconut cream; lovo,
The International Date Line passes through Fiji, which makes it a popular place for couples to ring in the new year

DIRECTIONS

- Fry garlic and onion for 1 minute on medium flame.
- Add chopped tomatoes and tuna and cook for another 1-2 minutes.
- Add lemon juice, evaporated milk, and chili sauce and toss well.
- Add cooked pasta and mix well.
- Sprinkle salt and black Pepper.
- Garnish with lemon wedges, fresh parsley, and green chili

Marshall Islands: Special salad

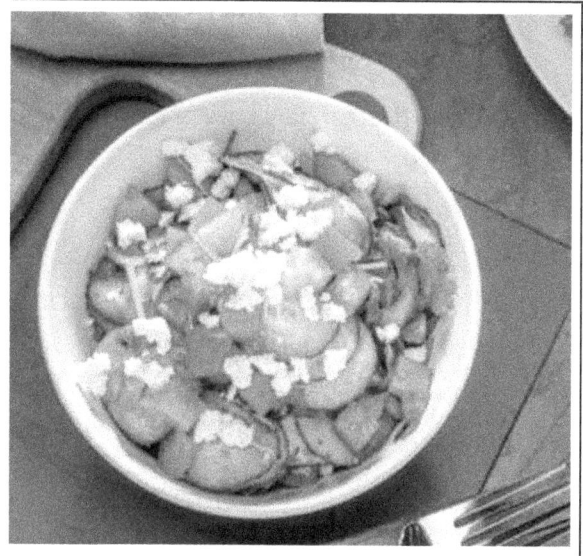

Marshall Islands

They are made up of more than 1,000 small islands and are part of the larger island group known as Micronesia.
Specialty foods of the Marshal Islands are fish, coconut, breadfruit, and Taro. And their ice tea, beer, coconut drinks are their traditional drinks.
Famous places include Kwajalein Atoll, Arno Atoll, and many other points. The atoll is home to a number of small islands, each with its own unique character and attractions.

INGREDIENTS

- Cucumber 1 thinly sliced
- Red Pepper 1 teaspoon.
- Green bell pepper 1 thinly sliced
- Yellow bell pepper thinly sliced
- Carrot 1 thinly sliced
- Mushrooms 12 ounces
- For dressing
- Vinegar
- Lime juice 2 tabspoon.
- Garlic powder 1/4 teaspoon
- Salt 1/4 teaspoon
- Black Pepper 1/4 teaspoon
- Cayenne Pepper 1/4 teaspoon
- Honey 1 teaspoon.
- Fresh parsley 2 tabs poon.

DIRECTIONS

- Whisk dressing ingredients.
- Mix all veggies plus mushrooms
- Pour dressing onto mixed veggies.
- Refrigerate for 1/2 hour and then serve.

Mali: Curry Noodle Salad

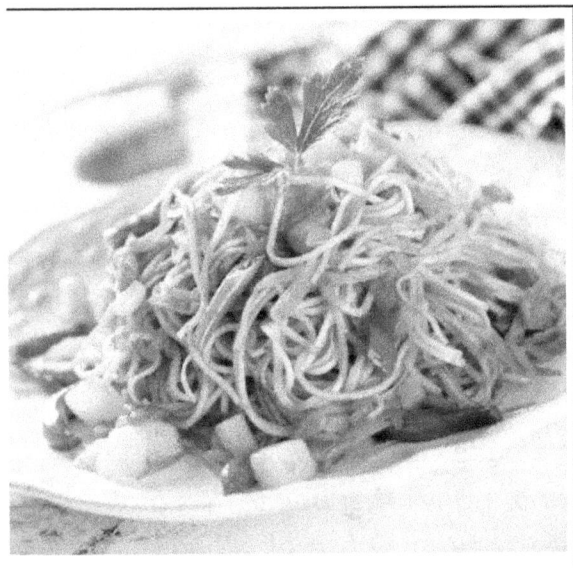

Mali

Mali is in West Africa. The capital city is Bamako.

Popular dishes include tieboudienne, which is a rice and fish stew, and mafé, which is a peanut-based sauce often served with meat or vegetables.

Their national drink is Kinkeliba

Mali is famous for its ancient cities, including Timbuktu and Djenné

Djenné is known for its Great Mosque, which is the largest mud-brick building in the world.

INGREDIENTS

- 500 grams' noodles screw or shells
- 1 tsp salt heaped
- 2-liter water boiled
- ½ red Pepper
- ½ green Pepper
- ½ yellow Pepper
- 1 onion
- 1 tbsp curry powder heaped
- 1 cup tomato sauce
- ½ cup vinegar
- ½ cup sunflower oil
- 1 cup sugar white or brown

DIRECTIONS

Dressing:
- Chop onion into fine cubes.
- Dice peppers into fine cubes.
- Add sugar.
- Add oil and vinegar.
- Add tomato sauce.
- Add curry powder.

Pasta:
- Boil in salted water until al dente.
- Strain and add to the dressing.
- Mix through thoroughly.

Mauritius: Mauritius salad

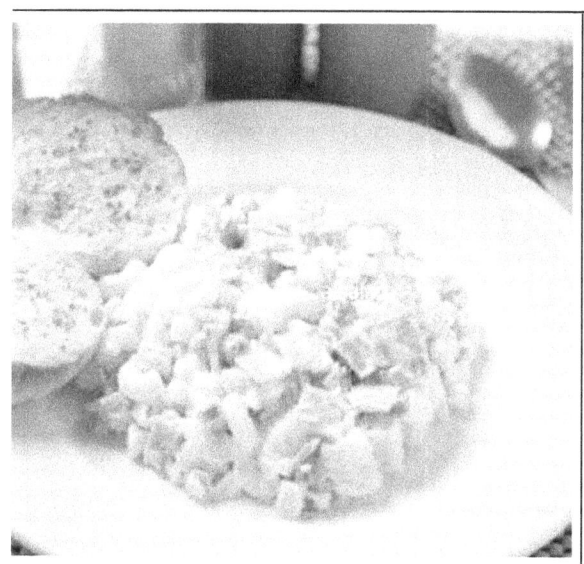

INGREDIENTS

- Boiled elbow macaroni 2 cups.
- Onions 1 chopped
- Celery stalks 2 chopped
- Carrot 1 chopped
- Green peppers 1 chopped.
- Red Pepper chopped 1
- Green bell pepper 1 chopped.
- For mayonnaise sauce.
- Mayonnaise 1 cup.
- Vinegar 4 tab spoon.
- Sugar 5 tab spoon.
- Mustard 2 teaspoon.
- Salt 1/2 teaspoon
- Crushed Black pepper 1/2 teaspoon.

Mauritius

The island is well known for its turquoise waters, white-sand beaches, lush vegetation, and crystal clear waters.

Mauritius is a beautiful destination for a vacation, and there are plenty of activities to keep you busy.

The island's main towns, such as Port Louis and Grand Port, are the best places to stay in Mauritius. There are also several resorts and villas available on the island. Mauritius is a great place to scuba dive, snorkel, and paddleboard. There are also a number of wildlife sanctuaries and interesting archaeological sites

DIRECTIONS

- Combine mayonnaise, mustard, sugar, salt, and Pepper. Mayo sauce is ready.
- Mix onion, celery stalks, carrot, green pepper, red pepper, green bell pepper, and elbow macaroni in a bowl.

Namibia: Namibian Salad

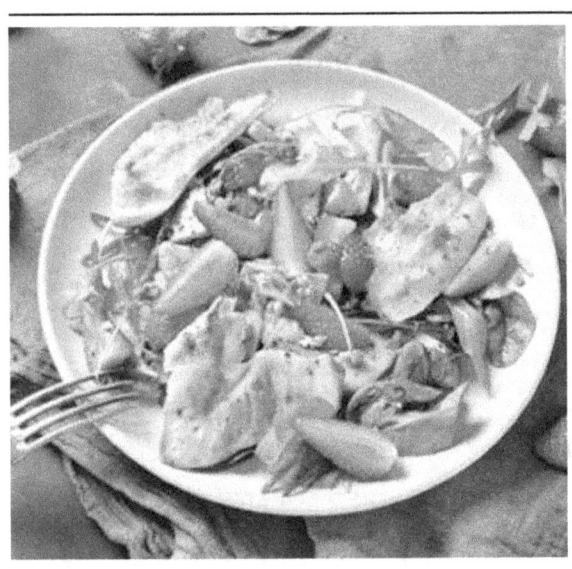

Namibia

Namibia is located in southern Africa and is bordered by Angola to the north and Zambia to the east. It is the smallest country in Africa by land area and has the highest population density of any country in the world. Namibia is home to numerous wildlife species, including lions, elephants, and hippos. The country is also known for its spectacular desert landscapes and rugged coastline. Namibia's rich cultural heritage includes traditional music, dance, and crafts.

INGREDIENTS

- Grilled chicken fillet 2 cut into small strips.
- Tie bow pasta boiled 2 cups
- Smoked paprika 2 teaspoons.
- Corn cobs remove silk 4.
- Garlic cloves 2
- Oregano 1 tab spoon
- Crushed red chili 1 teaspoon.
- Mayonnaise 1 cup.
- Lemon juice 2 tab spoon.
- Olive oil 1/2 cup.
- Honey 1 tab spoon.

DIRECTIONS

- Blend garlic, oregano chili, lemon juice, salt, and pepper.
- Stir in mayonnaise, honey, 4-tab spoon water, and 4-tab spoon oil.
- Blend until the mixture turns creamy and smooth.
- Mix chicken and all veggies.
- Toss well.

Niger: Niger pasta salad

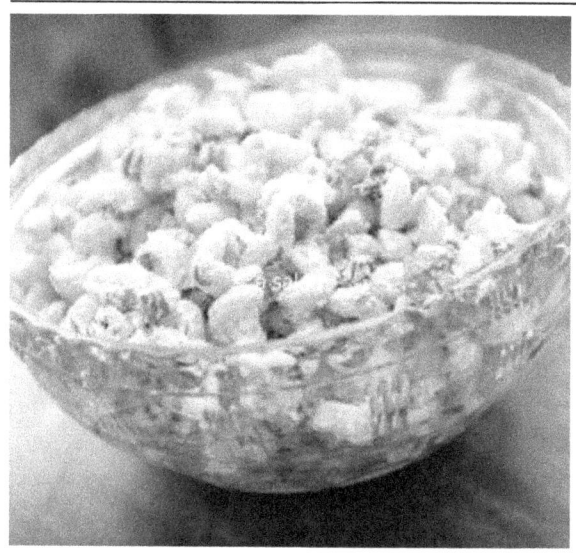

INGREDIENTS

- Boiled pasta 2 cups
- Cucumber chopped
- Tomato chopped
- Carrots chopped
- Boiled peas
- Sweet corn 1/2 cup.
- Ham 1 cup.
- Mayonnaise 1 cup
- Evaporated milk 1/4 cup
- Salt 1/2 teaspoon.

Niger

Niger is in Western Africa. The capital city is Niamey.

Nigerien cuisine is a blend of African, Arab, and French influences and the most popular beverage in Niger is tea, which is typically served sweetened and with mint.

Niger is known for its hospitality, with the people of Niger being known for their warmth and generosity. The country is famous for its diverse landscape, which includes the Sahara Desert in the north and the Niger River in the south. It is also known for its rich cultural heritage, with many different ethnic groups living in the country.

DIRECTIONS

- For sauce.
- Mix evaporated milk, salt, vinegar, and sugar in mayonnaise.
- Stir in all veggies plus ham strips.

Chad: Chad salad

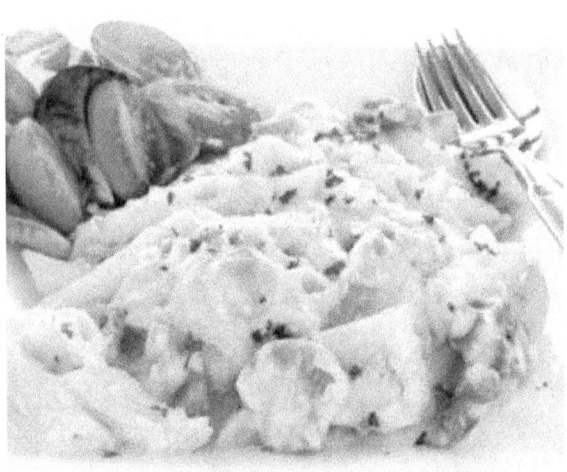

INGREDIENTS

- Boiled pasta 1 cup.
- Bananas 2
- Cucumber 2 chopped.
- Almonds 1/4 cup
- Raisins 1/4 cup
- Lemon juice 2 tabspoon.
- Olive oil 2 tabspoon
- Honey 1 teaspoon
- Cayenne Pepper
- Cumin seeds
- Coriander seeds

Chad

Chad is a landlocked country in Central Africa. Sudan borders it to the south and west, Cameroon to the northwest, and the Central African Republic to the northeast. The capital and largest city is N'Djamena.

Chad has a rich and diverse culinary culture, dishes such as kouttu a spicy meat stew and boule a meatball soup are popular.

One of the most common drinks is bouye, made from the fruit of the baobab tree, Tea and coffee

Chad is known for its vast and diverse landscapes, including the Sahara desert in the north, the Sahel region in the center, and the rainy forests in the south as well as largest wetlands in Africa,

DIRECTIONS

- Mix banana n Cucumber.
- Add dressing and toss well

Saskatchewan, Canada: Pasta Salad

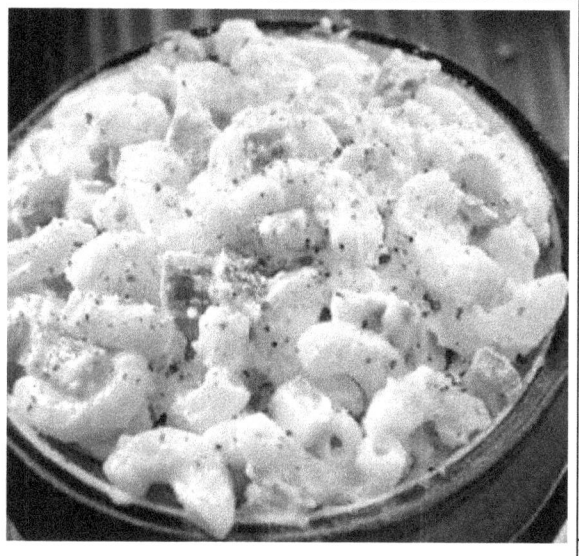

Saskatchewan, Canada

Saskatchewan is located in western Canada, bounded by the U.S. state of Montana to the south and east, Alberta to the southeast, and Manitoba to the north.

The popular foods are dumplings, borscht, and beet soup.

Drinks, Saskatchewan is home to a number of craft breweries producing a variety of beer styles, ales, lagers, and stouts.

INGREDIENTS

- Boiled pasta 1 cup.
- Bananas 2
- Cucumber 2 chopped.
- Almonds 1/4 cup
- Raisins 1/4 cup
- Lemon juice 2 tab spoon.

DIRECTIONS

-

Guadalajara, Mexico: Elbow Pasta Salad

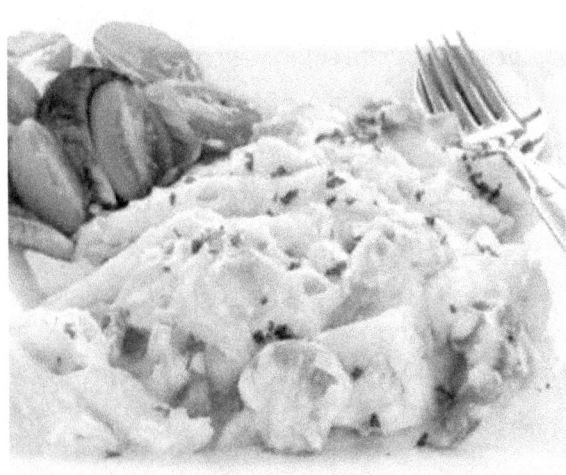

Guadalajara, Mexico

Guadalajara is a city located in the state of Jalisco in central Mexico.
The city is also famous for its delicious food, tortas ahogadas, birria, and pozole, rich history and vibrant arts and cultural scene. The city is known for its historical architecture and landmarks, including the Catedral de Guadalajara, the Teatro Degollado, and the Hospicio Cabañas.
Guadalajara host many major cultural events and festivals, such as the International Film Festival and the Guadalajara International Book festival.

INGREDIENTS

- Dry elbow macaroni boiled 2 cups
- Red onion chopped soak in water for 5 minutes and then drained.
- Tomato chopped 1
- Celery diced 1 chopped.
- Fresh parsley 2 tabspoon

For dressing:

- Mayonnaise 1/2 cup
- Sour cream 3 tabspoon.
- Vinegar 2 tabspoon
- Sugar 1 tabspoon
- Mustard 1/2 teaspoon.
- Salt 1/2 teaspoon
- Crushed black pepper 1/4 teaspoon

DIRECTIONS

- Whisk all dressing ingredients.
- Mix all veggies plus pasta
- Stir in mayo dressing and mix well.
- Garnish with fresh parsley.

Huatulco, Mexico: Pasta Salad

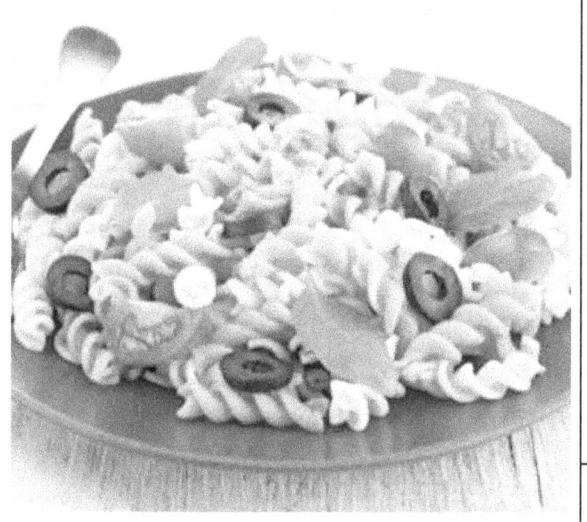

Huatulco, Mexico

Huatulco is a beautiful place to visit in Mexico. It is nestled in the mountains and has stunning ocean views for, hiking, biking, swimming and kayaking.
The town also has a few restaurants, bars, and souvenirs shops.
Huatulco is a great place to relax and soak up the Mexican culture.

INGREDIENTS

- Pasta boiled 2 cups
- Butter 2-tab spoon.
- Tomato 2 chopped
- Chervil 1 teaspoon
- Chives chopped 1 teaspoon.
- Green onions 1 chopped
- Tarragon chopped 1 teaspoon.
- Radishes 2 sliced
- Feta cheese crumbled 1/4 cup.
- Celery leaves for garnishing.

Dressing:
- Olive oil 2-tab spoon
- Lime juice 2-tab spoon.
- Dijon mustard 1 teaspoon.
- Sugar 1 teaspoon.
- Salt 1/2 teaspoon.

DIRECTIONS

- Add pasta, butter, tarragon, chives, chervil, parsley, salt, black pepper.
- Let it rest for 15 minutes.
- Then add radishes, onions, cheese, tomatoes, dressing, and toss well.
- Garnish with celery leaves and serve.

Las Vegas Nevada: Vegetable Pasta Salad

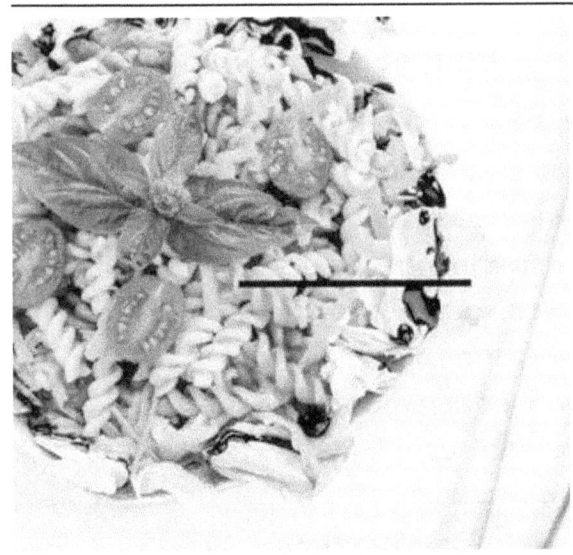

INGREDIENTS

- Macaroni boiled 2 cups
- Bell pepper 1 chopped
- Lettuce leaves 2
- Tomato 2 chopped
- Cheese grated 1/4 cup.
- Potato boiled 1
- Chicken boiled and shredded 1 cup
- Mayonnaise 1 cup
- Cream 2 tabspoon
- Olive oil 2 tabspoon.
- Mustard powder 1
- pinch.
- Hot sauce 1 teaspoon.
- Sugar 1 teaspoon.
- Crushed black pepper 1/4 teaspoon.

Las Vegas Nevada

Las Vegas is a city in the U.S. state of Nevada. The city is located in the Las Vegas Valley, on the southern end of the Las Vegas Strip. It is known for its vibrant nightlife, entertainment, and gambling. Their waffles, pork, watermelon, lobster roll, pie, and cocktails are really famous in the town. Las Vegas is often referred to as the "Entertainment Capital of the World" because of its casinos, hotels, museums, art galleries, and other cultural attractions as well as its fine dining, shopping, and other luxury amenities.

DIRECTIONS

- Mix olive oil, mayonnaise, cream, mustard powder, black pepper, sugar, hot sauce, boiled chicken, macaroni, cheese, bell pepper, and potato in a bowl.
- Chill for 1/2 hour and then serve.

Charleston, West Virginia: Pasta Salad

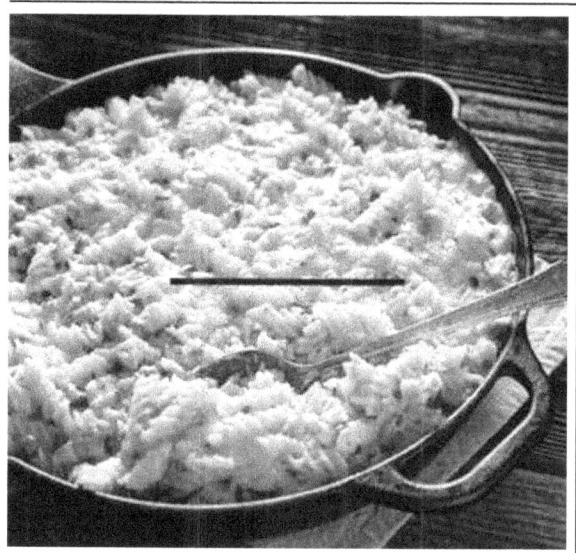

Charleston, West Virginia

Charleston, West Virginia, is located in the state's southwestern corner. Some popular dishes and local specialties in Charleston include pepperoni rolls, ramp dishes, and coal-fired pizza. If you're looking to try something truly unique, you might want to try a "float", a local specialty that combines ice cream and soda. Charleston is a thriving small city with a vibrant arts and culture scene. The city has several historical sites, including the National Military Park at Manassas, the restored Governor's Palace, and the Kanawha Canal.

INGREDIENTS

- Penne pasta boiled 2 cups.
- Zucchini sliced 1/2
- Cherry tomatoes 2 cut in half.
- Bell pepper 1 chopped
- Scallions sliced 1
- Olives 10
- Parmesan cheese 1/2 cup
- Fresh basil 2 tabspoon.
- Pepperoni sliced 1/4 cup
- Dressing
- Olive oil 2 tabspoon
- Lime juice 2 tabspoon
- Salt 1/2 teaspoon
- Sugar 1 teaspoon
- Oregano 1/4 teaspoon.

DIRECTIONS

- Mix dressing ingredients.
- Combine all vegetables, pour dressing, and mix well

Ukraine: Ukrainian pasta salad

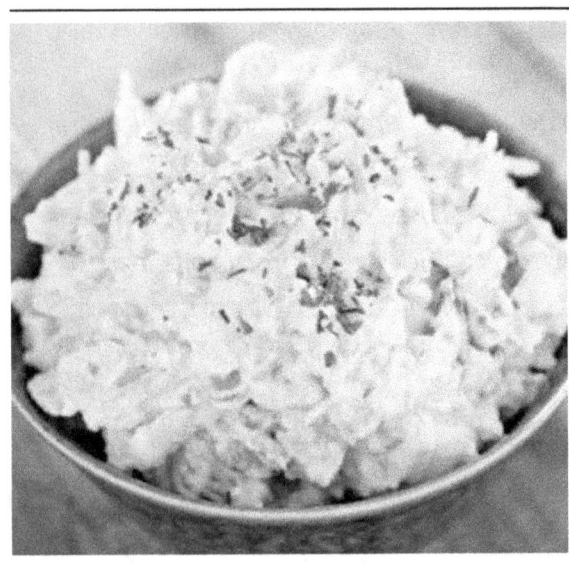

INGREDIENTS

- Pasta boiled 1 cup
- Cucumber 1 diced
- Tomato 1 chopped
- Red onion 1 chopped
- Dill chopped 1/4 cup
- Olive oil 2-tab spoon.
- Salt 1/4 teaspoon
- Black pepper 1/4 teaspoon

For mayo sauce.
- Mayonnaise 1 cup
- Evaporated milk 1 /4 cup
- Vinegar 1-tab spoon
- Brown sugar 1/2 teaspoon.

Ukraine

Ukraine is a country in Eastern Europe. Russia borders it to the north, Belarus to the east, Poland to the south, and Hungary and Romania to the west.

Ukraine is known for its delicious and hearty cuisine. Their borscht, dumplings, bread, patties, and stews are flavorful. Additionally, Ukraine is known for its fruit wines and liqueurs, such as cherry wine and the honey-flavored liqueur known as medovukha. Some of the things that Ukraine is famous for include its beautiful architecture, folk art and traditions, and delicious food. The country is also known for its natural beauty, with the Carpathian Mountains, the Black Sea, and the Dnieper River being some of its most notable natural attractions.

DIRECTIONS

- Mix all vegetables and pasta.
- Mix mayo sauce ingredients.
- Pour mayo sauce n to salad veggies

Romania: Romanian salad

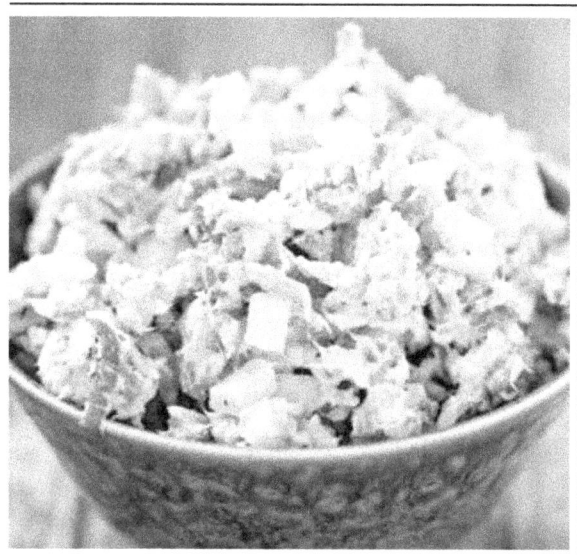

INGREDIENTS

- Pasta boiled 2 cups.
- Red onions chopped 1
- Hard-boiled eggs 2
- Celery 2 sticks chopped
- Green bell pepper 1 sliced.
- Red bell pepper 1 sliced

For mayo sauce

- Mayonnaise 1 cup
- Mustard 1/2 teaspoon.
- Basil 1/2 teaspoon
- Oregano 1/2 teaspoon
- Red chili powder 1/2 teaspoon.
- Crushed Black pepper 1/2 teaspoon.

Romania

Romania is in Central and Eastern Europe Some popular dishes in Romania include mici (grilled minced meat rolls), sarmale (stuffed cabbage rolls), and papanasi (cheese-filled pastries topped with sour cream and jam). Romanian food is often hearty and filling, with a focus on meat, potatoes, and vegetables.
Romania is known for its wine and plum brandy, called tuica.
Plan to trip to the Carpathian Mountains,The city of Sighisoara, where the famous Dracula (Vlad the Impaler) was born.

DIRECTIONS

- Mix all veggies.
- Whisk mayo sauce ingredients.
- Add veggies and boiled pasta to mayo sauce
- Serve immediately.

Netherlands: Netherland salad

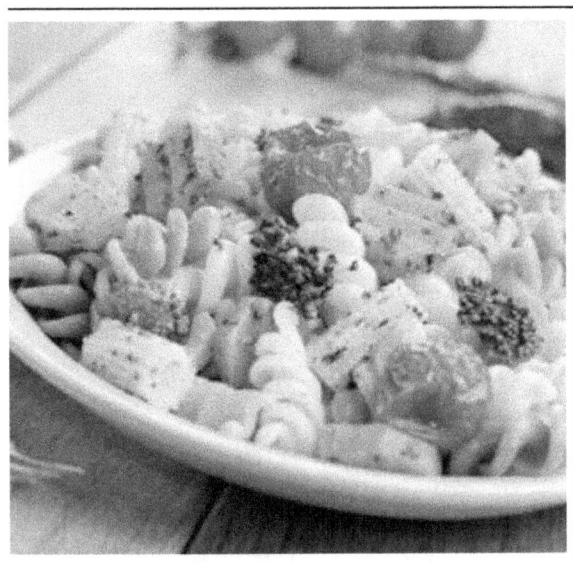

Netherlands

The Netherlands is in Western Europe. It is the most populous country in the European Union.
The Netherlands borders Belgium, Germany, and the North
The official language of the Netherlands is Dutch, but there are also major languages spoken, including Afrikaans, Frisian, and Amharic.
The Netherlands has a rich cultural history, with many famous painters, musicians, and writers.
The country is also known for its tulips, cheese, and windmills.

INGREDIENTS

- Fusilli 1 cup
- Sun-dried tomatoes
- Rocket or Arugula green leafy veggie use for salads. 1 cup
- Artichoke 1/4 cup
- Shallot 1/4 cup.
- Walnut 2-tab spoon.

DIRECTIONS

- Mix all vegetables plus walnuts and olive oil

Austria: Austrian Salad

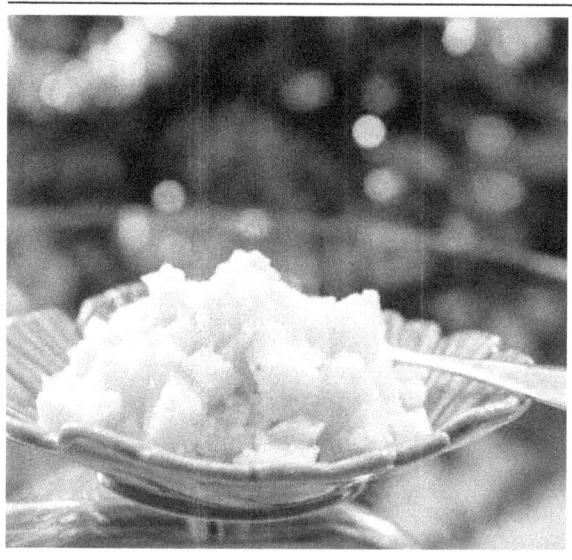

Austria

Austria, is in Central Europe. The capital city is Vienna, a popular tourist destination, known for its museums, theaters, and concert halls.

Popular foods in Austria include schnitzel (breaded and fried veal), gulasch (beef and vegetable stew), and knödel (dumplings). Austria is also known for its wines pastries and desserts, such as strudel (pastry filled with fruit or cheese) and Sachertorte (a chocolate cake)

INGREDIENTS

- 2 tbsps pumpkin seed
- 5 ozspickled pumpkin (canned or from a jar)
- 7 ozschicken aspic
- 1small red onion
- 1 bunchradish
- 2tomatoes (about 150 grams)
- 2 tbspsapple cider vinegar
- 2 tspsmustard
- salt
- peppers
- 4 tbspspumpkin seed oil

DIRECTIONS

- Lightly toast pumpkin seeds in a dry frying pan. Remove from heat and let cool slightly.
- Drain pumpkin.
- Cut aspic into 1 cm (approximately 1/4-inch) wide strips.
- Peel onion and cut into very thin slices.
- Rinse radishes and cut into thin slices. Rinse tomatoes and cut out stem ends. Cut tomatoes into slices.
- Coarsely grind cooled pumpkin seeds in a mortar. Combine pumpkin seeds with vinegar, mustard, salt and pepper. Stir to combine. Stir in pumpkin seed oil.
- Rinse lamb's lettuce and arugula and spin dry.
- Toss greens with 3/4 of the pumpkin dressing and place on a plate. Garnish with all of the remaining ingredients and drizzle with the remaining dressing. Serve.

Serbia: Serbia salad

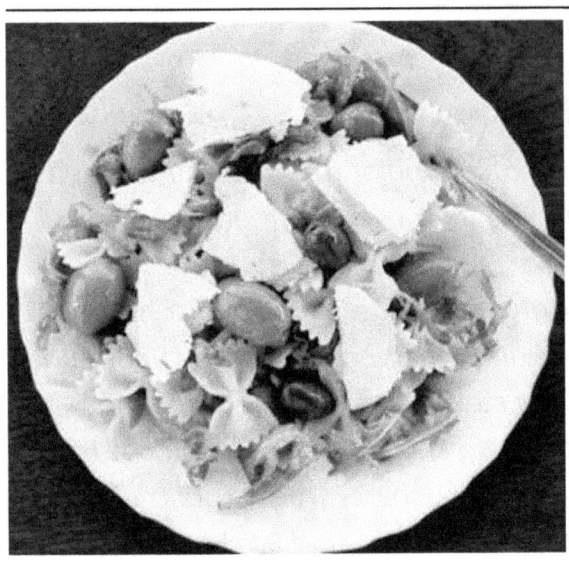

Serbia

Serbia is located in the Balkan Peninsula, bordering Bosnia. The capital and largest city is Belgrade.

Serbia has a rich cultural heritage. Its traditional music, dance, and theater are well-known around the world.

It is also having a diverse natural environment, with mountains, rivers, and forests.

INGREDIENTS

- Boiled pasta 1 cup
- Cucumber 3 cut with peels
- Tomatoes 3 diced
- Red onion 1 chopped
- Red bell pepper 1 chopped.
- Feta cheese grated 1/2 cup.
- Olive oil 2-tab spoon
- Lemon juice 2-tab spoon
- Dried oregano 1/2 teaspoon
- Salt 1/4 teaspoon
- Black Pepper 1/4 teaspoon.

DIRECTIONS

- Mix all salad ingredients with boiled pasta and enjoy this mouth-licking salad

Section iv

Legumes, Meat or Grains-Mixed Salads

There are unlimited creative ways to prepare salad using grains or legumes. One great way to mix things up is to create a mixed salad. Here are some tricks for you on how to make a healthy and delicious mix of grains and legumes

- *Start by selecting a variety of grains and legumes to mix together. This can include quinoa, bulgur, couscous, farro, and lentils.*
- *Next, choose a salad dressing or sauce to go with the mix. Options include tahini dressing, a vinaigrette, or a simple olive oil and vinegar mixture.*
- *Finally, mix everything and serve.*

Guatemala: Special Cucumber, bean, watermelon, and feta salad

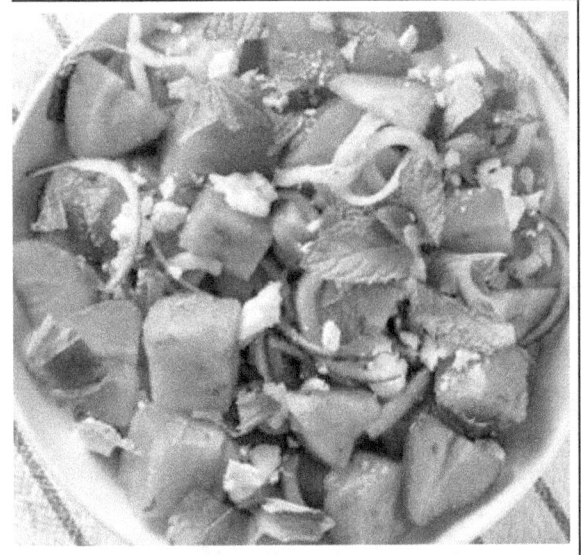

Guatemala

Guatemala is in Central America. The capital and largest city is Guatemala City. Guatemala has a diverse culture that reflects its indigenous Mayan heritage as well as Spanish colonial influences. Chuchitos, Tortillas, and Tamales are some famous foods as well as a variety of tropical fruits, including pineapples, mangoes, papayas, and avocados. Guatemala is known for its natural beauty, including volcanoes, rainforests, beaches and archaeological site - ancient Maya city of Tikal,

INGREDIENTS

- White beans 1 cup
- Cucumber 1 peeled and sliced
- Watermelon 1 cup.
- Olive oil 1/4 cup
- Vinegar 2 tabspoon.
- Mint chopped 1 tabspoon.
- Feta cheese 1/4 cup.

DIRECTIONS

- Mix white beans, Cucumber, and watermelon
- Add olive oil, vinegar, chopped mint, salt, black pepper and mix well.
- Top with crumbled feta cheese, and enjoy!

Peru: Chickpeas, spinach, and tomato salad

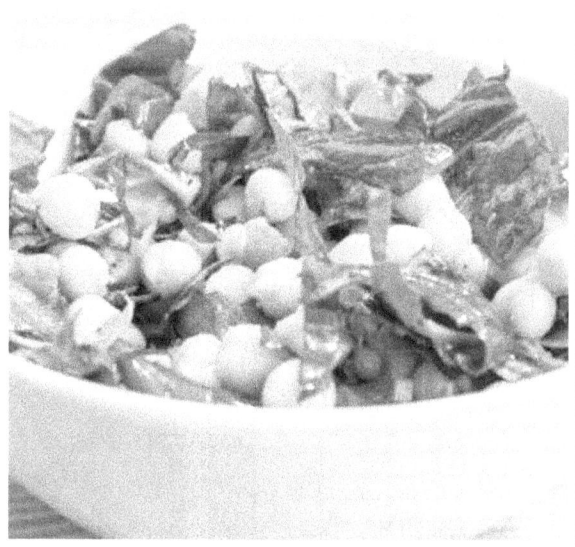

INGREDIENTS

- Canned chickpeas 1 drain water and set aside.
- Canned tuna 1 small can.
- Cucumber peel and diced.
- Spinach boiled 1 cup.
- Tomato 2 diced.
- Salt 1/4 teaspoon
- Crushed black pepper. 1/4 teaspoon.

Peru

Peru, located in western South America. The capital and largest city is Lima, and the official language is Spanish.

Peruvian cuisine is known for its mix of indigenous, Spanish, and Asian flavors and ingredients. Some popular Peruvian dishes include Lomo saltado, Causa, rellena, and Ceviche.

Peru is also known for its diverse range of fruits, including avocados, papayas, mangos, and passionfruit. The country is also a major producer of coffee, cocoa, and various types of grains and vegetables.

Peru has a rich and diverse history, with influences from indigenous cultures, the Inca Empire, and Spanish colonization. The country is home to many ancient ruins and archaeological sites, including the famous Inca citadel of Machu Picchu.

DIRECTIONS

- Mix all ingredients.
- Chill for 2 hours and then serve.

Suriname: Special Fava bean salad

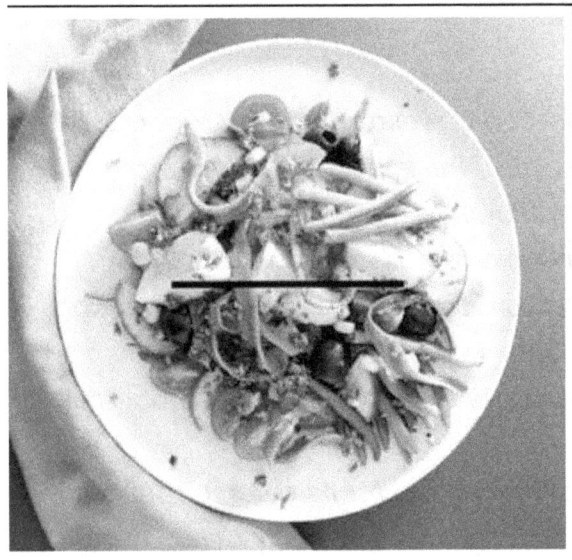

INGREDIENTS

- Fava beans boiled 1 cup
- Fresh peas cooked 1/2
- Lettuce leaves 3
- Hard-boiled eggs 2
- Parmesan cheese 1/2 cup
- Olive oil 2tabspoon
- Dijon mustard 1 teaspoon.
- Lemon juice 1 tab spoon.

Suriname

Suriname is a country located in northern South America with the capital and largest city being Paramaribo, and the official language is Dutch.
Suriname is home to a variety of ecosystems, including rainforests, swamps, and savannas. Roti, sate, chicken or beef curry, and moksi meti are some famous cuisines of this country. The country's coastal location means that seafood is also an important part of the local diet, with fish and shellfish being commonly consumed. Suriname is also home to a number of beautiful beaches, including Galibi Beach, where visitors can go turtle watching and see the leatherback turtles that come to nest. As well as its rich natural resources and its rainforests., diamonds, and other minerals.

DIRECTIONS

- Mix fava beans, hard-boiled eggs, and peas.
- Add lemon juice, olive oil, Dijon mustard, and mix all ingredients.

meat or grains-mixed salads

Saint Lucia: Lentil salad with olives and tuna

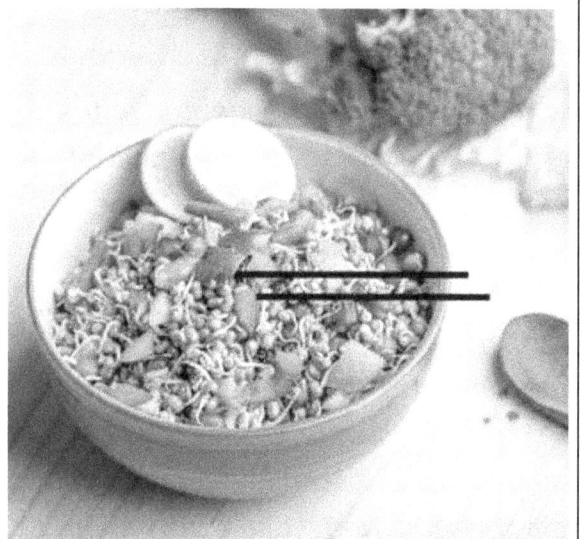

INGREDIENTS

- Canned lentils 1 cup
- Black olives 10
- Roasted bell pepper 1/2
- Tuna cooked

Saint Lucia

Saint Lucia is a small island country situated in the eastern Caribbean Sea, just east of the Dominican Republic. The island is about 120 miles long and 50 miles wide, with a population of just over 103,000 people. Saint Lucia is made up of three main islands - Saint Lucia, Soufriere, and Gros Islet - and a number of smaller islets.

The capital city is Castries. Saint Lucia is a Commonwealth realm; its monarch is Queen Elizabeth II.

The economy is dependent on agriculture, with significant production of bananas, sugarcane, and tobacco.

DIRECTIONS

- Mix all ingredients until all are well combined.

Aruba: Shrimp and chickpea salad

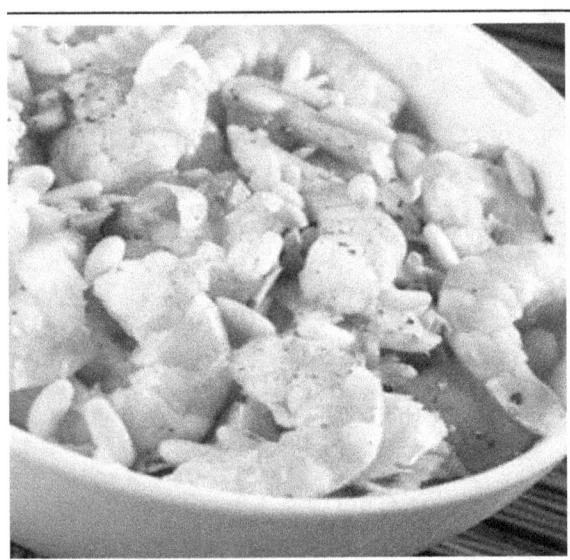

Aruba

Aruba is a Caribbean island located in the southern Caribbean Sea, off the coast of Venezuela. The capital and largest city is Oranjestad.

The island is known for its seafood. Popular Aruban dishes include keshi yena, funchi, saffraanbollen, and karkoeri as well as the coconut milk mixed drinks.

Aruba is known for its beautiful beaches, with crystal-clear waters and white sandy shores and a variety of plant and animal species.

INGREDIENTS

- Spinach 1 cup
- Shrimps 1 cup.
- Canned Chickpeas.1
- Diced melon 1 /2 cup.
- Salt 1/2 teaspoon

DIRECTIONS

- Mix all veggies.
- Drizzle olive oil.
- Season with salt and pepper.

United States Virgin Islands: American pasta and bean salad

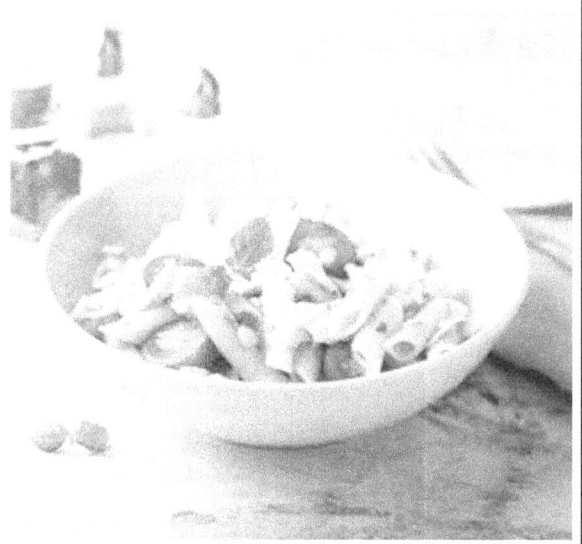

INGREDIENTS

- Elbow macaroni 1 cup
- Boiled kidney red beans 1 cup dry elbow macaroni, cooked, rinsed, and drained
- Red onion 1 chopped, soak in water for 5 minutes to remove its bitterness.
- Celery 1 diced.
- Parsley 1-tab spoon
- Mayonnaise 1 cup
- Dijon mustard 1/2 teaspoon.
- Sugar 1/2 teaspoon
- Apple cider vinegar 2-tab spoon.
- Sour cream 3-tab spoon.
- Crushed black pepper 1/4 teaspoon.

United States Virgin Islands

The United States Virgin Islands (USVI) are a group of islands located in the Caribbean Sea, east of Puerto Rico. The capital and largest city is Charlotte Amalie.
Conch fritters, roti, and Johnnycakes are mostly preferred foods.
The USVI are composed of three main islands: St. Croix, St. John, and St. Thomas. The USVI are known for its beautiful beaches, crystal-clear waters, and tropical climate. Tourist love to visit this beautiful place. It is home to several resorts, & Spa.

DIRECTIONS

- Mix mayonnaise, sour cream, Apple cider vinegar, sugar, salt and pepper.
- Add red onions, celery, macaroni, red, beans and toss well.
- Garnish with fresh parsley and enjoy this delicious. Salad.

Antigua and Barbuda: Cucumber, beans and feta cheese salad

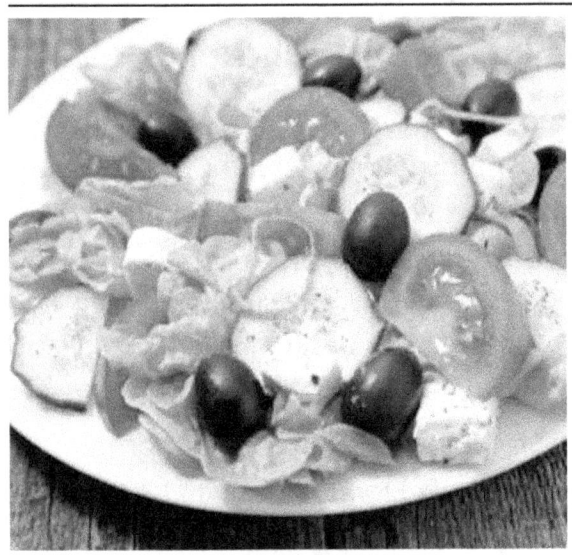

INGREDIENTS

- White beans 1 cup
- Soybeans 1/2 cup
- Cucumber 1 peeled and sliced
- Watermelon 1 cup.
- Olive oil 1/4 cup
- Vinegar 2 tabspoon.
- Mint chopped 1 tabspoon.
- Feta cheese 1/4 cup.

Antigua and Barbuda

Antigua and Barbuda is a country of two islands Antigua and Barbuda, located in Caribbean Sea. The country is part of the Lesser Antilles and is located east of Puerto Rico and the Virgin Islands. Its capital is St. John's, which is located on Antigua.

Fish and lobster are commonly caught and eaten in the country. Popular dishes in Antigua and Barbuda include "ducana," a sweet potato pudding, and "breadfruit cou-cou," which is made with breadfruit and cornmeal.

Antigua and Barbuda is known for its beautiful beaches, music, festivals, and rum, which is often used in cocktails like the "Antiguan Sunset."

DIRECTIONS

- Mix white beans and Cucumber.
- Add olive oil, vinegar, chopped mint, salt, black pepper and mix well.
- Top with crumbled feta cheese, and enjoy!

Dominica: Dominican salad

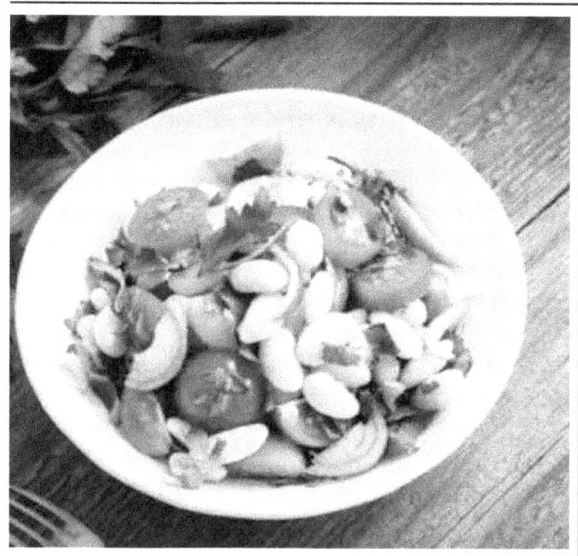

Dominica

It is the smallest country in the Caribbean and has a population of just over 77,000. Dominica is known for its stunning natural beauty, including its dramatic mountains and rainforest-covered coastline.

The country is also home to many interesting historical sites, including the ruins of an old sugar plantation.

Dominica's rich culture is known for its traditional music and dance. It is a great place to visit, and its natural beauty and culture make it a unique destination.

INGREDIENTS

- Yellow onion, 1 sliced thinly,
- Fava beans boiled and peeled 2 Cups.
- Bacon 1cup.
- Red bell pepper 1 chopped.
- Apple cider vinegar 2 tabspoon
- Salt 1/2 teaspoon.
- Crushed black pepper 1/4 teaspoon.
- Fresh parsley 2 tabspoon.

DIRECTIONS

- Browning bacon
- Heat 1 tabspoon butter in a non-stick pan.
- Add bacon and cook until the edges are browned. It will take 1 minute to change the color.
- Add onions and cook until onions become soft and translucent.
- Stir in red bell pepper and Fava beans and continue stirring until it is heated well.
- Add salt, vinegar, black pepper and cook for a while.
- Sprinkle some fresh parsley on top

The Maldives: Maldeev tuna salad mashuni

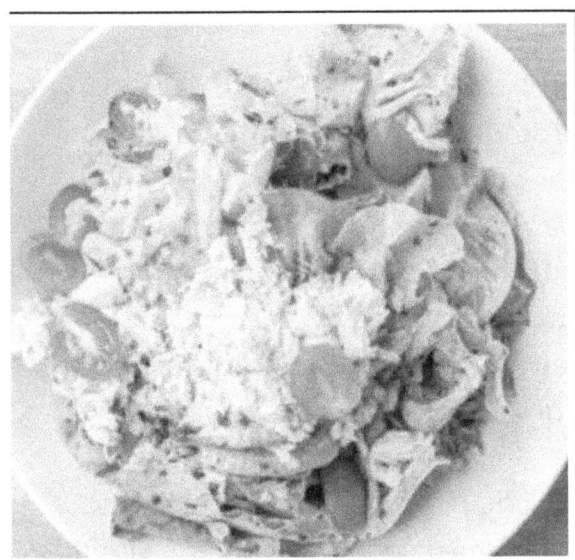

The Maldives

The Maldives is a small island nation located in the Indian Ocean.
It is made up of 26 atolls and is located in the southwest of India and Sri Lanka. The capital of the Maldives is Male.
Fish and seafood are a staple in many dishes as well as rice and coconut. Popular fruits are mangoes, papayas, and coconuts.
Fun actives include water sports and scuba diving.

INGREDIENTS

- Onion 1 sliced
- Chili 1 chopped
- Canned tuna 1 cup
- Fresh grated coconut 3 tabspoon
- Curry leaves 1
- Lime 1/2

DIRECTIONS

- Drain water from the tuna fish can.
- Add onion, chili, tuna fish, and coconut in a bowl; squeeze lime juice and mix well with light hands.
- Enjoy with flat bread roshi.

Asia

Nepal: Nepali salad

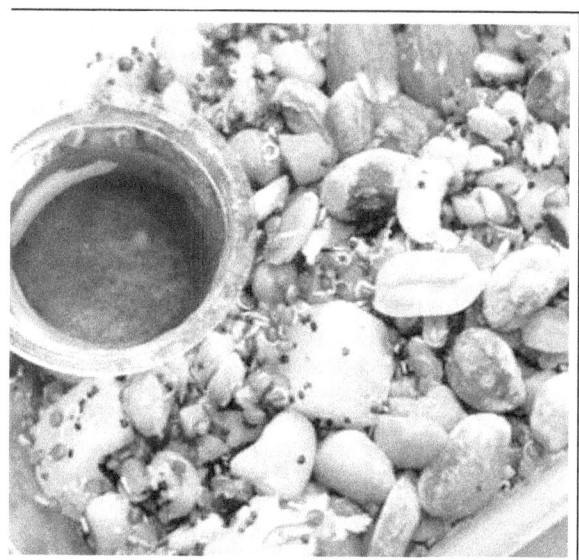

INGREDIENTS

- Roasted peanuts 1 cup.
- Chilli pepper 1 thinly sliced.
- Garlic 2 cloves chopped.
- Green onion 1 chopped.
- Onion chopped 1/4 cup.
- Tomato 1 chopped.
- Ginger 1/2 inch thinly sliced.
- Cumin powder 1/4 teaspoon.
- Red chili powder 1/4 teaspoon.
- Lime juice 1 tabspoon.
- Fresh cilantro 2 tabspoon.
- Mustard oil 1 tabspoon.

Nepal

Nepal is a small, mountainous country located in South Asia, between India and China.

Nepal is known for its stunning natural beauty, with the Himalayas running through the country and known for the world's highest peak, Mount Everest.

Daalbhat, momo, Thukpa, and tea are some famous foods and beverages.

Nepal has a rich cultural heritage, with a number of important cultural and historical sites, including the Kathmandu Valley. The country is also home to a number of festivals and events throughout the year, including Dashain, the biggest festival in Nepal, which is celebrated with family gatherings, feasts, and the exchange of gifts.

DIRECTIONS

- Mix roasted peanuts, garlic cloves, green onion, Chile pepper, and sliced ginger
- Add chili powder, cumin powder, and salt to the bowl with the rest of the ingredients and mix well.
- Heat mustard oil in a pan, add tomato and crushed red chili. sauté for 1 minute until the tomatoes get soft
- Add turmeric and cook for a few seconds.
- Pour this cooked mixture onto salad ingredients and mix well.
- Add lime juice, salt and mix well.
- Garnish with fresh parsley

Sri Lanka: Sri Lankan Salad

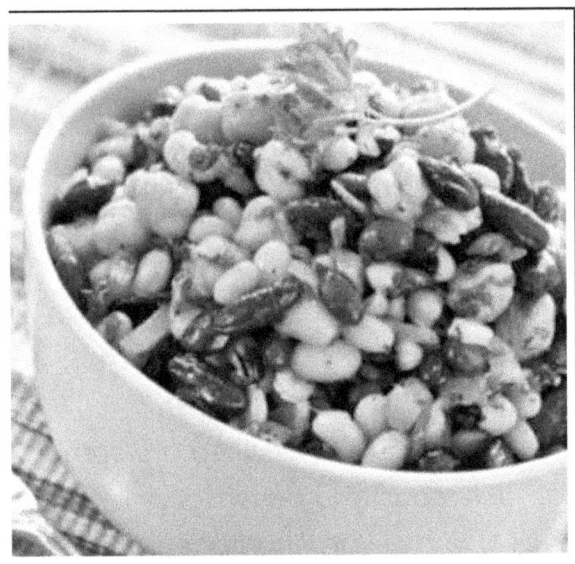

Sri Lanka

Sri Lanka is a tropical island nation located in the Indian Ocean with the capital city, Jayawardenepura Kotte.

This country is known for its stunning beaches, beautiful temples and palaces, and rich wildlife.

Coconut water is a popular drink in Sri Lanka, and can be found at many street stalls and markets. Curry, rice, and roti are popular dishes.

Sri Lanka is a popular tourist destination, with visitors coming to see the country's natural beauty and cultural attractions, beautiful beaches, stunning wildlife, and picturesque landscapes, including tea plantations, national parks, and waterfalls.

INGREDIENTS

- Dried Black Eye Beans boiled 1 cup
- Red kidney beans cooked 1 cup
- Dried Marrowfat Peas 1/2 cup.
- Green onion 1 chopped
- Red chili pepper 1 chopped
- Fresh dill 2 tablespoon chopped
- Fresh parsley 2 tabspoon chopped.
- Mango 1 chopped.
- Olive oil 2 tabspoon
- Lime zest 1 teaspoon
- Lime juice 1 tabspoon.
- Salt 1/2 teaspoon.

DIRECTIONS

- Add mixed beans, green onions, dill, mango, red chili pepper, lime zest and mix well
- Add lime juice, olive oil, salt, black pepper, and toss well.
- Garnish with fresh parsley.

Iran: Iran legume salad

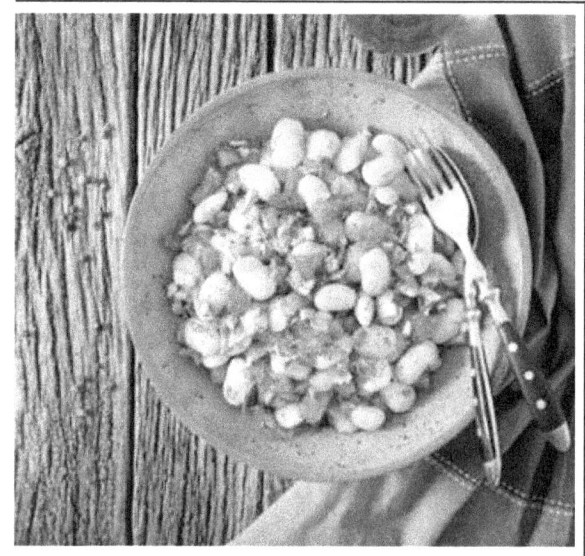

INGREDIENTS

- Mixed beans from can 2 cups drain water and set aside
- Onion 1 chopped
- Tomato 1 chopped
- Fresh parsley 1/4 cup.
- Red Sumac 1 teaspoon
- Olive oil 1-tab spoon.
- Lemon juice 1-tab spoon
- Pomegranate juice 1 tabspoon.
- Salt 1/4 teaspoon
- Crushed black pepper 1/4 teaspoon.
- For garnish.
- Walnuts and hard-boiled eggs.

Iran

The second-largest country in the Middle East, Iran. The capital city is Tehran.

Iran has a long and rich history, and is known for its cultural and historical sites, including ancient ruins, palaces, and mosques.

Their kebabs, rich dishes, and soups are very popular foods. Tea and coffee are refreshing drinks.

Iran has a rich cultural heritage, with a number of important cultural and historical sites, including the ancient city of Persepolis, the Tehran Museum of Contemporary Art, and the Golestan Palace in Tehran. The country celebrates many festivals and events throughout the year.

DIRECTIONS

- Add mixed beans, onion, parsley, and tomato in a bowl.

Asia

Jordan: Jordanian Salad

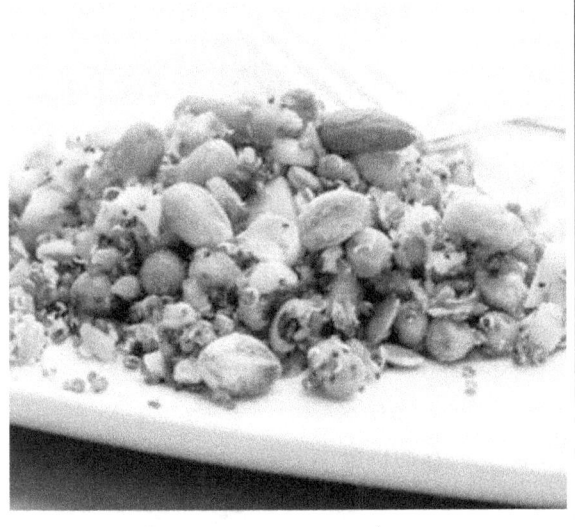

INGREDIENTS

- Peas boiled 1 cup
- Courgettes chopped 2
- Baby gem lettuce 1 chopped
- Onion 1 chopped
- Garlic cloves 3
- Olive oil 4-tab spoon
- Artichokes 2 chopped
- Red Sumac 1 teaspoon.
- Salt 1/4 teaspoon.
- Labneh hang yogurt 1/4 cup.

Jordan

Jordan is a country in the Middle East. It is located on the East Bank of the Jordan River. Amman is the capital of Jordan. Jordanian cuisine is a mix of Middle Eastern and Mediterranean flavors, and it is known for its diverse and flavorful dishes like falafel, shawarma, hummus, and kebabs. Some popular drinks in Jordan are Arabic tea, Arak, and Jallab.

The country is known for its rich cultural heritage, including ancient sites such as Petra, Jerash, and the Dead Sea. Jordan is also home to a number of nature reserves and protected areas, such as Wadi Rum and the Dana Biosphere Reserve.

DIRECTIONS

- Heat oil, add onion and garlic cloves, and cook until onions get soft.
- Cut courgettes and artichokes into slices, add some salt, mix and set aside.
- Mix soft-cooked onions, courgettes, peas and artichokes, red Sumac, salt and pepper
- Stir in hang yogurt and mix well.
- Serve and enjoy!

Palau: Legume salad

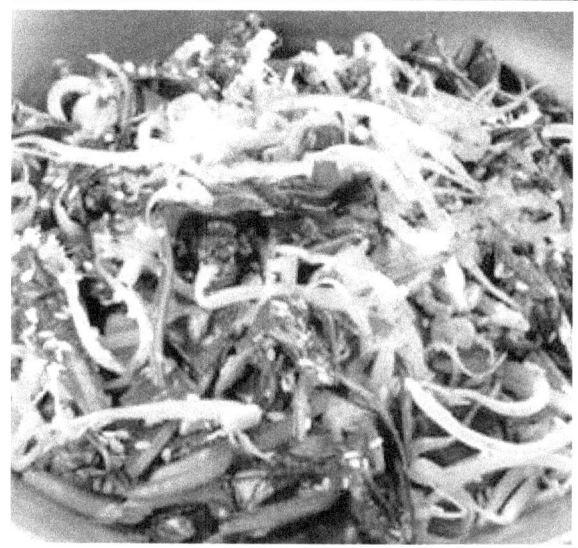

INGREDIENTS

- Red kidney beans 1 cup.
- Celery 2 stalks chopped.
- Tomato 1 chopped
- Bean sprouts 1/4 cup.
- Hard-boiled eggs 2
- For dressing
- Salad oil 2-tab spoon
- Vinegar 1-tab spoon
- Mayonnaise 1/4 cup.
- Salt 1/4 teaspoon
- Crushed black pepper 1/4 teaspoon

Palau

A nation of small Islands, located in the western Pacific Ocean, Palau. It is made up of more than 500 islands and is part of the Micronesia region.
The capital city of Palau is Ngerulmud, transferred from Koror city.
Fish, Sago, Taro, Tea and coffee are their famous cuisines and beverages.
The people of Palau have a rich cultural heritage and are known for their traditional music, dance, and art.
Palau is known for its natural beauty, with crystal clear waters and coral reefs that are home to a rich variety of marine life. The country is also home to a number of protected areas, including the Rock Islands in the Southern Lagoon.

DIRECTIONS

- Mix oil, vinegar, mayonnaise, salt, and pepper in a bowl.
- Mix all veggies, drizzle dressing, and toss well.

Papua New Guinea: Special lettuce and bean sprouts salad

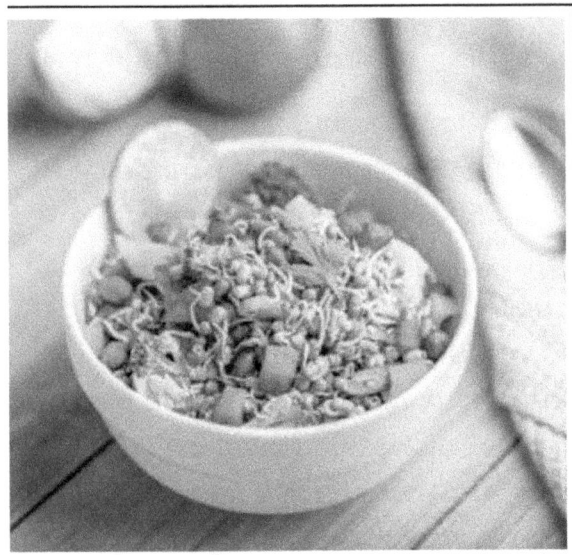

INGREDIENTS

- Lettuce 1 head small
- Shallots 3 chopped
- Salt
- Black pepper 1/4 teaspoon
- Fresh bean sprouts 1 and 1/2 cup
- Olive oil 2 tab spoon
- Lemon juice 2 tab spoon

Papua New Guinea

Papua New Guinea is a located in the southwestern Pacific Ocean, east of Indonesia and north of Australia. It is in the eastern half of the island of New Guinea, the world's second-largest island. The capital city of Papua New Guinea is Port Moresby.

Papua New Guinea is also known for its seafood, particularly its prawns, crab, and lobster. Drinks in Papua New Guinea include a variety of locally produced beers and liqueurs, as well as imported spirits and wine. Papua New Guinea is known for its adventure tourism opportunities, including rafting and diving. The country is also known for its birds of paradise, tree kangaroos, and marsupial moles, as well as a variety of reptiles and amphibians

DIRECTIONS

- Mix all vegetables
- Add lemon juice, olive oil and toss all ingredient.

Samoa: Decorated salad

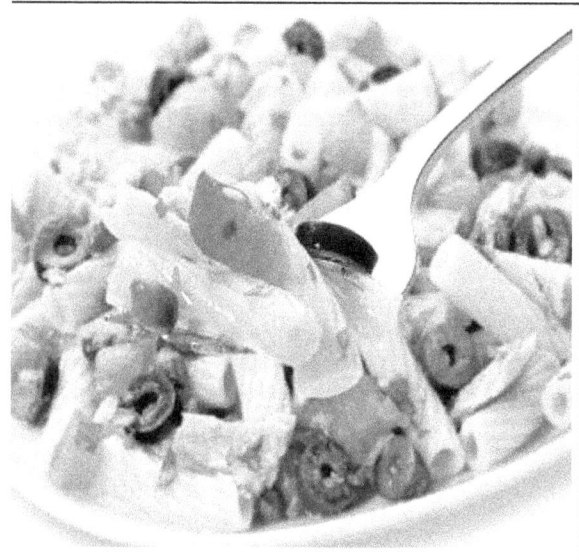

Samoa

Samoa, also known as the Independent State of Samoa, is a country located in the South Pacific Ocean, east of Tonga and west of American Samoa.
The capital city of Samoa is Apia.
Staple foods in Samoa include taro, yams, and bananas, which are often served with fish, chicken, pork, or beef. Coconut is also a common ingredient in Samoan cooking, and is used in a variety of dishes and drinks. Samoa is made up of two main islands, Upolu and Savai'i, and several smaller islands. The country is also a popular destination for adventure travelers, with a range of activities available including surfing, snorkeling, and hiking.

INGREDIENTS

- Green beans boiled sliced 1/2 cup.
- Onion 1 chopped.
- Carrot boiled 1, peeled, and sliced.
- Potatoes 2 boiled
- Hard-boiled eggs 2 sliced in rings.
- Radish 1 sliced.
- Tomato cut in wedges.
- Capers 1 tab spoon
- Olivc 10 sliced.
- Anchovy fillets 4
- Salt 1/4 teaspoon
- Crushed black pepper 1/4 teaspoon.

For dressing:

- Olive oil 2 tab spoon
- Lemon juice 2 tab spoon
- Mustard powder 1/2 teaspoon.
- Salt 1 pinch.
- 1 ice cube

DIRECTIONS

- Blend all French dressing ingredients.
- Mix green beans, carrot, onion, potato, tomato, capers, chives, black olives.
- Decorate with radish and onion rings.
- Drizzle dressing over the veggies and refrigerate for 1/2 hour.

Senegal: Senegalese Salad

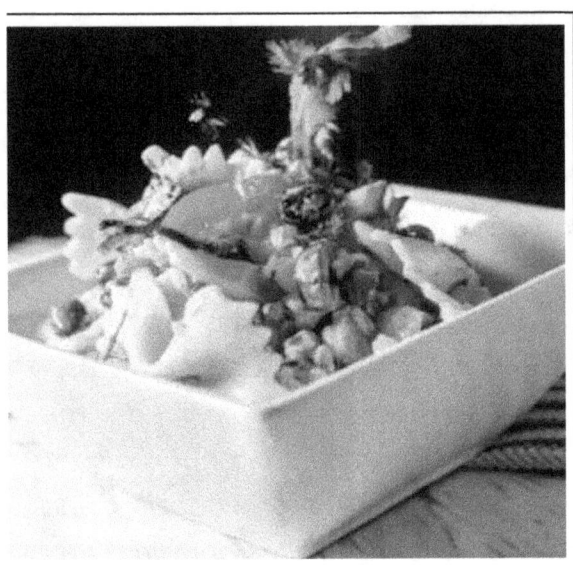

INGREDIENTS

- Rotini Boma pasta 2 cups.
- Red kidney beans 1 cup
- Green bell pepper 1 chopped
- Red bell pepper 1 chopped
- Red onion 1 chopped.
- Garlic cloves 5 chopped
- Celery 1 cup
- Sugar 1 tabspoon.
- Crushed red Pepper 1/2 teaspoon.
- Curry powder 1 tabspoon.
- Turmeric 1/4 teaspoon.
- Salt 1/2 teaspoon.
- Black Pepper 1/4 teaspoon.

Senegal

Senegal, is located on the western coast of Africa with the capital city of Senegal is Dakar.
The Atlantic Ocean lies to the west of Senegal.
Seafood is particularly important in Senegalese cuisine, with fish, shellfish, and octopus being widely consumed.
Bissap, a drink made from the hibiscus flower, is popular as well.
Senegal is home to a number of beautiful beaches and natural areas, including the Niokolo-Koba National Park.
Also known for its rich art and craft traditions, including wood carving, pottery, and textiles.

DIRECTIONS

- Boil pasta in some salt and water
- Drain and let it cool down
- Stir in pasta and beans to veggies.
- Enjoy!

Seychelles: Seychelles salad

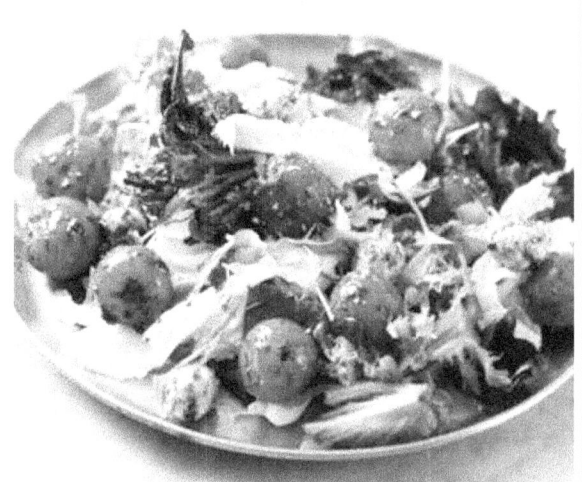

INGREDIENTS

- Cherry tomatoes 2 diced
- Cucumber 2 sliced cut with peels.
- Red onion 1 chopped
- Fresh cilantro 1/4 cup.
- Jalapeno remove seeds and then diced 1
- Salt 1/4 teaspoon
- Crushed Black pepper 1/4 teaspoon.
- Lemon juice 2 tabspoon.
- Olive oil 2 tabspoon.

Seychelles

The Seychelles is an archipelago of 115 islands located in the Indian Ocean and its capital city is Victoria.

Seychellois dishes include octopus curry, seafood stew, and coconut cakes.

The Seychelles is also known for its tropical fruits, such as mangoes, papayas, and pineapples, which are often used in desserts and juices.

The Seychelles is also home to a number of unique species of flora and fauna, including the giant tortoise and the coco de mer, a type of palm tree that produces the largest seed in the world.

It is a popular tourist destination, attracting visitors from around the world with its stunning natural beauty and rich cultural heritage.

DIRECTIONS

- Add red onions, cherry tomatoes, fresh cilantro, chopped jalapeno,
- Season with salt and black Pepper.
- Add lemon juice and toss all ingredients.

Somalia: Somalian salad

Somalia

A nation situated in the Horn of Africa, Somalia. Its capital city is Mogadishu. Somali cuisine uses lots of spices, such as cumin, coriander, and cardamom, with lamb, goat, and seafood.

In Somalia, a popular traditional drink is called "sahwa," which is made from roasted and ground barley. As well as "shaah," which is made from camel's milk.

The natural beauty of Somalia's landscapes, including its long coastline, white sandy beaches, and lush forests.

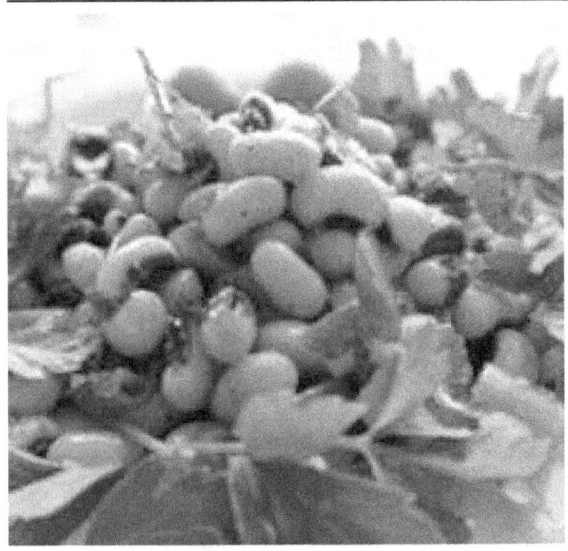

INGREDIENTS

- Black-eyed peas.1 cup.
- Cherry tomatoes 3 sliced
- Cucumber 1 thinly sliced.
- Red bell pepper 1 chopped.
- Red onion 1 chopped.
- Pearled barley 1 cup.
- Tamarind sauce of any good brand1/2 cup.
- Olive oil 2 tab spoon.
- Lime juice 1/4 cup.
- Honey 1teaspoon.
- Salt 1/2 teaspoon.

DIRECTIONS

- For making the dressing, mix tamarind sauce, lime juice, onions, salt, and honey until all well combined.
- Add salt in the water and let it boil.
- Add barley and cook for 25 minutes on medium flame.
- Add hot cooked barley in the dressing.
- Soak until barely absorb all the liquid.
- It will take maximum 5 minutes.
- Add cucumbers, black eyed peas, bell pepper, parsley, and tomatoes in a bowl and toss well.
- Chill for 1 hour.
- Sprinkle some fresh parsley and avocado slices on the salad before serving

Burundi: Mixed beans and corn salad

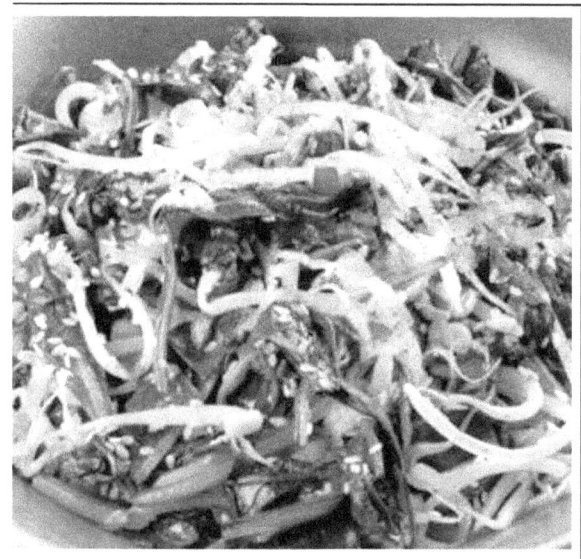

INGREDIENTS

- Boiled corn 1 and 1/2 cup
- Red kidney beans 1 and 1/2 cup
- Soybeans 1/4 cup
- Butter beans 1/4 cup
- Celery 2 stalks chopped
- Shallots 1/4 cup chopped
- Red onion 1 chopped.
- Red bell pepper 1/4 cup chopped.
- Fresh parsley 2 tab spoon chopped.
- Olive oil 2 tab spoon
- Lime juice 2 tab spoon
- Salt 1/2 teaspoon
- Black pepper 1/2 teaspoon.

Burundi

Burundi is a landlocked country located in East Africa and its capital city is Bujumbura. Burundian culture is a blend of African and European influences, and the country has a rich tradition of music, dance, and storytelling.

Burundian cuisine uses ingredients, such as beans, cassava, and sweet potatoes, and often includes dishes made with goat, chicken, and fish.

In Burundi, a popular traditional drink is called "urwarwa," which is made from fermented banana or plantain juice.

Burundi is famous for its stunning natural beauty, including its lush forests, rolling hills, and picturesque lakes and rivers.

DIRECTIONS

- Mix all ingredients, add olive oil, lime juice, salt, and pepper, and toss well.
- Garnish with fresh parsley.

Tunisia: Tunisian salad

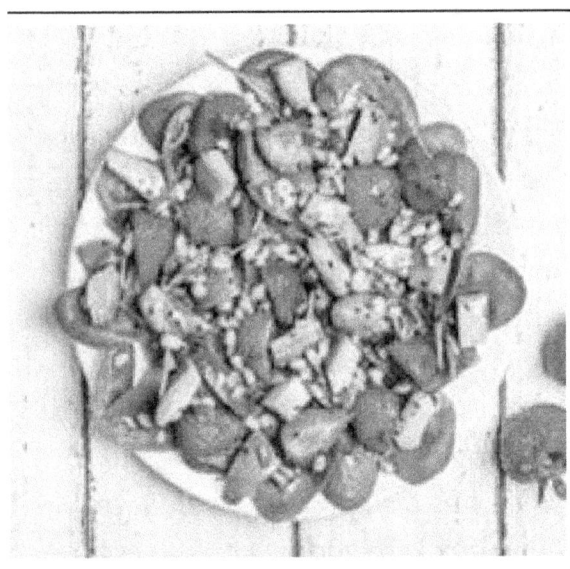

Tunisia

Tunisia is located in North Africa, on the Mediterranean Sea. The capital and largest city is Tunis. The country is made up of three main islands, which are connected by a bridge. This country is known for its rich history and cultural heritage.

Couscous (a traditional Tunisian dish), Harissa, Stew, and Brik are famous cuisines of Tunisia. Some famous beverages are coffee, mint tea, beer, and Almaza.

It is known for its stunning beaches, ancient ruins, and beautiful landscapes.

Some of the popular tourist attractions in Tunisia include the Medina of Tunis, the Bardo Museum, which houses a collection of Roman mosaics and other artifacts, and the El Djem Amphitheatre, a well-preserved Roman ruin.

INGREDIENTS

- Yellow Bell Pepper 1 chopped
- 1 Red Onion 1 chopped.
- Roma tomatoes 2 chopped.
- 1 Lemon 1 cut into halves.
- Carrots 2 chopped
- Green chili pepper 1 chopped
- Black Olives 10 sliced.
- Baby Spinach 1 cup boiled.
- Radishes 2 sliced
- Garlic Cloves 2 chopped
- Red Pepper Flakes 1/2 teaspoon
- Green Lentils 1 cup boiled.

DIRECTIONS

- Mix all veggies plus lentils in a bowl.
- Season with red chili pepper, salt, and black Pepper. Add lemon juice, and enjoy!

British Columbia, Canada: British Columbia salad

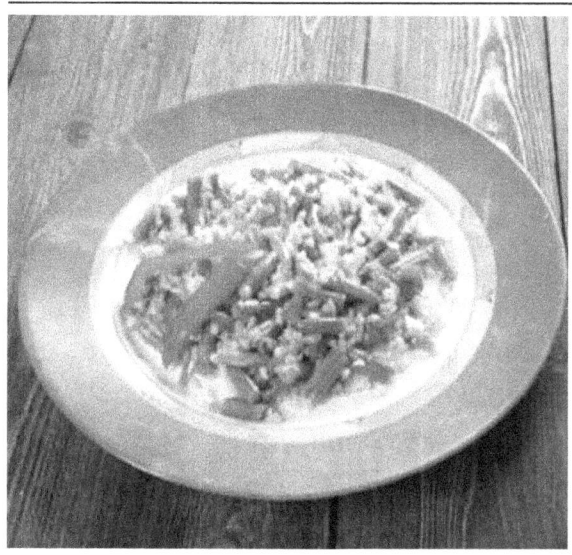

INGREDIENTS

- Green beans 1 cup
- Soya beans 1/2 cup.
- Cucumber 3 chopped
- Roasted sesame seeds 2 tabspoon
- Hot sauce 1 teaspoon
- Dressing.
- Vegetable oil 1/2 cup
- Rice vinegar 1/4 cup.
- Honey 1 teaspoon.
- Salt 1/4 teaspoon.
- Black Pepper 1/4 teaspoon.

British Columbia, Canada

British Columbia is a beautiful place to visit. The province is located in Canada and has a population of about 4.5 million. The province's diverse geography is home to many interesting things to explore. Visitors enjoy the natural beauty, culture, the lakes and rivers of the province. The province is the hub of a variety of different mountains and forests. Some popular dishes and drinks include Spot prawns, Pacific oysters, Ice wine, Craft beer, cider, and coffee

DIRECTIONS

- Mix all ingredients and enjoy this healthy bean salad.

Mexico City, Mexico: Mexico bean salad

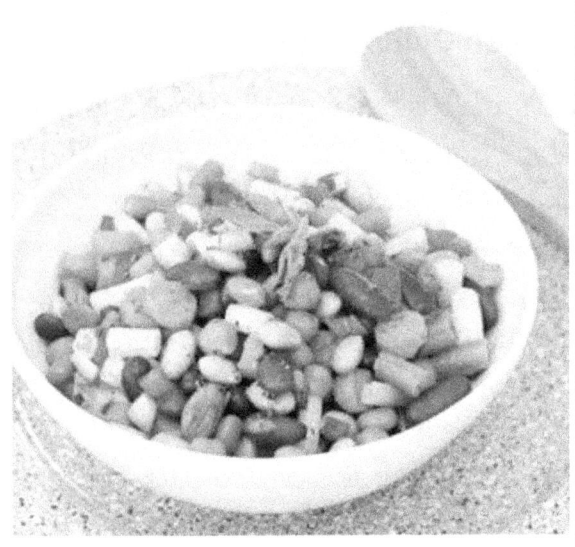

Mexico City, Mexico

Mexico City is included in one of the world's most populous and largest cities. The city is famous for its rich history and culture, as well as its vibrant nightlife and extensive shopping districts. The city is also renowned for its extensive public transportation system, which makes it easy to get around. Popular foods and drinks of Mexico are Burritos, Enchiladas, and Quesadillas, as well as Mexican beer and cocktails

INGREDIENTS

- Red beans 1 cup
- Black beans 1 cup
- Bell pepper 1 chopped.
- Red onion 1 chopped.
- Jalapeno 2 chopped
- Fresh cilantro 1/4 cup.
- For dressing.
- Vinegar 1/2 cup
- Olive oil or salad oil 4 tabspoon.
- Roasted cumin 1 teaspoon.
- Salt 1/4 teaspoon.
- Crushed Black pepper 1/4 teaspoon.

DIRECTIONS

- Whisk all dressing ingredients.
- Mix all vegetables plus beans.
- Pour dressing.
- Refrigerate for 30 minutes

San Cristobel de las Casas, Mexico: San Cristobel de las Casas, Mexico Salad

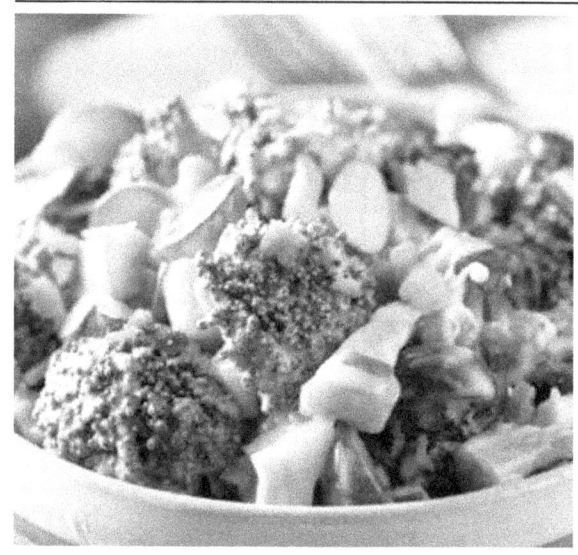

INGREDIENTS

- Boiled tie bow or any pasta you like boiled 2 cups
- Broccoli 1 cup
- Lettuce leaves 3
- Tomatoes 2 chopped.
- Garlic 1/2 teaspoon chopped.
- Mixed herbs 1 teaspoon
- Salt 1/4 teaspoon.
- Crushed Black pepper 1/2 teaspoon.
- Olive oil 1 tabspoon
- Lemon juice 1-tab spoon.
- Vinegar 1-tab spoon.
- Honey (optional) 1 teaspoon.

San Cristobel de las Casas, Mexico

San Cristobel de las Casas, is in the southern state of Chiapas, it is one of the oldest and most important of the Mexican colonial towns, with narrow streets and whitewashed buildings.

The town is also known for its richly decorated churches, including the Basilica of Our Lady of the Assumption, considered one of Mexico's most important colonial churches.

Mole, Tamales, Pozole, Mezcal, and tortillas are known for their diverse and flavorful cuisine. Horchata is a sweet, refreshing drink made from rice, almonds, and cinnamon, and is often served cold over ice.

DIRECTIONS

- San Cristobal mixed All the Vegetables Together.
- Add Salad dressing.

Detroit Michigan: Detroit Special corn salad

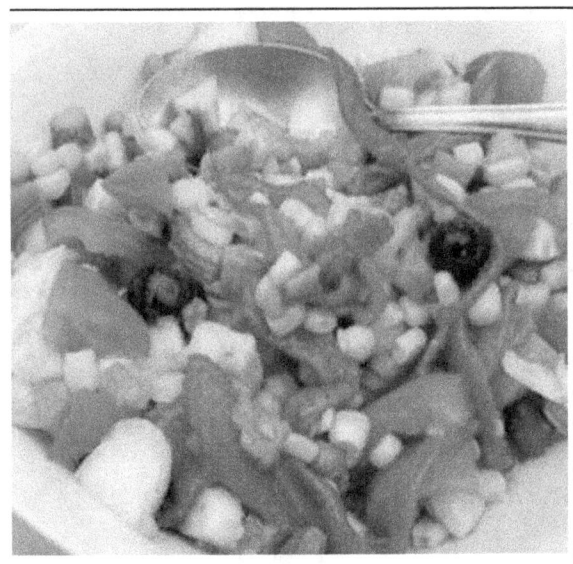

INGREDIENTS

- Corn boiled 1 cup
- Tomato 1 chopped
- Cucumber 2 thinly sliced
- Green bell pepper ½ chopped. Jalapeno 1 chopped
- Parsley ¼ cup chopped
- Lime 2
- Vinegar 2 tab spoon.
- Salt
- Black Pepper to taste

Detroit Michigan

Detroit is a city in Michigan. It is the biggest city in the state, the largest in the mid west and the fourth largest in the United States. Antoine de la Mothe Cadillac, a French trader, and explorer, founded Detroit on July 24, 1701.

It is known for its rich history, cultural legacy, popular food are Coney dogs, Detroit-style pizza, dumplings, sausages, and pepperoni. The city is also known for its music scene, with a number of music venues and festivals throughout the year, including the Detroit Jazz Festival and the Movement Electronic Music Festival.

DIRECTIONS

- Add all veggies in a bowl
- Add salt, black pepper, lime juice, vinegar, salt, and black pepper and mix until all well combined.

Phoenix, Arizona: Phoenix, Arizona salad

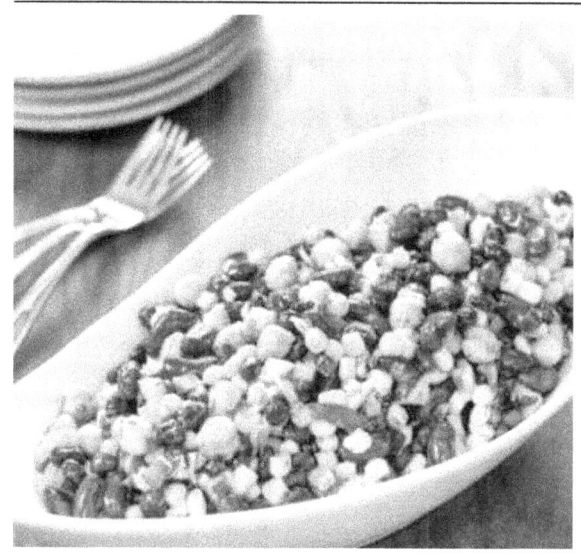

INGREDIENTS

- Boiled corn 1 cup
- Red kidney beans boiled 1 cup
- Cabbage shredded 1 and 1/2 cup
- Green bell pepper 1 chopped
- Red bell pepper 1 chopped
- Tomato 2 chopped.
- Carrot 1 chopped.

For dressing

- Sour cream or hung curd 1 cup
- Canola or olive oil 2 tab spoon
- Lemon juice ¼ cup.
- Salt ¼ teaspoon
- Sugar 1/2 teaspoon.
- Dried oregano ½ teaspoon
- Thyme ½ teaspoon.
- Black Pepper ¼ teaspoon.

Phoenix, Arizona

Phoenix is situated in Maricopa County, Arizona, and is the state's capital.
It is known for its warm, dry climate and sunshine, making it a popular destination for vacationers.
Some popular dishes and drinks include Sonoran hot dogs, Mexican food, BBQ, green chile, and prickly pear drink
Natural attractions, including the Sonoran Desert and the Grand Canyon and a wide range of outdoor activities, such as hiking, biking, and golfing.

DIRECTIONS

- Mix all dressing ingredients with sour cream or hung curd. Give it a nice stir.
- Add all veggies in this special dressing and combine well.

Slovenia: Slovenian Salad

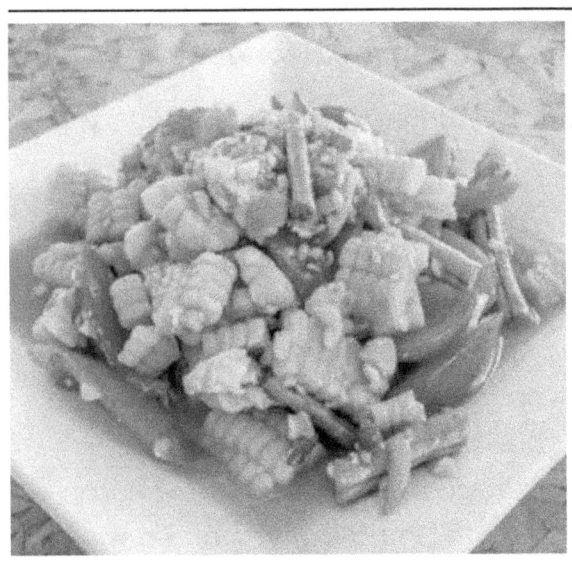

INGREDIENTS

- Corn sweet 1 can use 1 and 1/2 cup.
- Garlic cloves 2
- Cucumber 1 thinly sliced.
- Cheese 2 tabspoon
- Yogurt 2 tabspoon
- Feta cheese crumbled 1/4 cup
- Red pepper roasted and peeled 1
- Olive oil 2 tab spoon
- Salt 1/4 teaspoon
- Crushed black pepper 1/4 teaspoon.
- Fresh dill or parsley 2 tab spoon.

Slovenia

Slovenia is a landlocked country in the central Balkans region.
The capital and largest city is Ljubljana.
Their sweet bread, dumplings, sausages, and pastries are some of the popular foods.
Slovenia is also known for its wine, especially its white wine.
It is also known for it natural beauty and outdoor activities, such as hiking, skiing, and mountain biking in the Julian Alps and the Karst Plateau.

DIRECTIONS

- Remove water from the corn can.
- Add Cucumber, garlic, and mix.
- Whisk cheese yogurt, feta cheese, salt, and pepper and add to veggie bowl.
- Add olive oil and toss well.
- Garnish with fresh dill or parsley.

Latvia: Latvian Salad

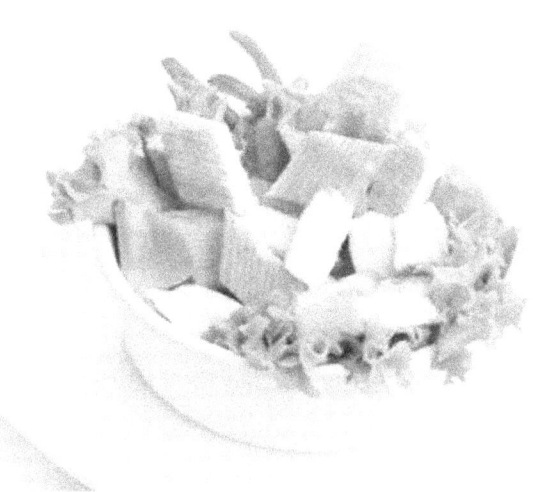

Latvia

Latvia is a small Baltic country on the eastern coast of the Baltic Sea.
The capital of Latvia is Riga. This country has cold winters and mild summers.
Latvian cuisine is a blend of influences from its neighbors, including Russia, Germany, Sweden, and Poland.
Popular Latvian dishes include Sklandrausis, Kāpostu zupa, Kvass, and Rupjmaize.
Latvia is known for its beautiful natural landscapes forests & lakes wine, folk traditions, dance, handicrafts, such as woven baskets and pottery.

INGREDIENTS

- Boiled and shredded chicken 1 and 1/2 cup.
- Crab sticks 3 cut into small cubes.
- Avocado peeled and cut 1
- Green onion 1 chopped
- Red pepper 1 chopped.
- Lettuce leaves 3
- Bean sprouts 2 cups.
- Celery chopped 2 stalks.
- Dill chopped 2 tabspoon
- Basil 2 tabspoon.
- Parsley 2 tabspoon
- Salt 1/4 teaspoon
- Crushed black pepper
- Yogurt 1 cup
- Lemon juice 2 tabspoon
- Sugar or honey 1 tabspoon.

DIRECTIONS

- Mix yogurt, lemon juice, honey, salt, black pepper, and dill in a bowl.
- Mix chicken crab sticks, bean sprouts, green onions, celery, pepper, and
- basil
- Presentation
- Place lettuce leaves onto a serving platter.
- Add mixed salad. Pour dressing. Garnish with parsley.
- Chill and serve.

Estonia: Salad "Chick-chick"

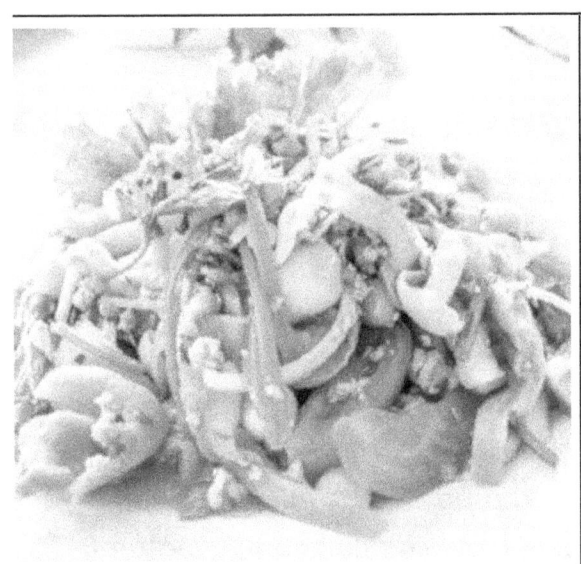

INGREDIENTS

- Fried chicken fillet, cut into thin strips. 1 cup
- Pickled mushrooms 1/4 cup
- Canned peas 1 cup
- Horseradish grated 2 tab spoon
- Cheese 1 cup grated
- Cream 1/2 cup
- Salt 1/4 teaspoon
- Crushed black pepper 1/4 teaspoon
- Walnuts crushed 1/4 cup.

Estonia

Estonia is a small country on the eastern coast of the Baltic Sea.
The capital of Estonia is Tallinn.
It is known for its beautiful natural landscapes, including forests, lakes, and islands.
Oats and barley dessert, sausages, peas and pork soup are famous Estonian cuisines.
Estonia is also known for its beers, such as Saku and A. Le Coq, and for its spirits, such as Vana Tallinn and Kannu Kukk.
The country is also home to a number of cultural and historical landmarks, such as Tallinn's Old Town, the Toompea Castle, and the Kadriorg Palace. National Park

DIRECTIONS

- Mix all ingredients.
- Chill for 1/2 hour and then serve.

Malta: Mediterranean Salad

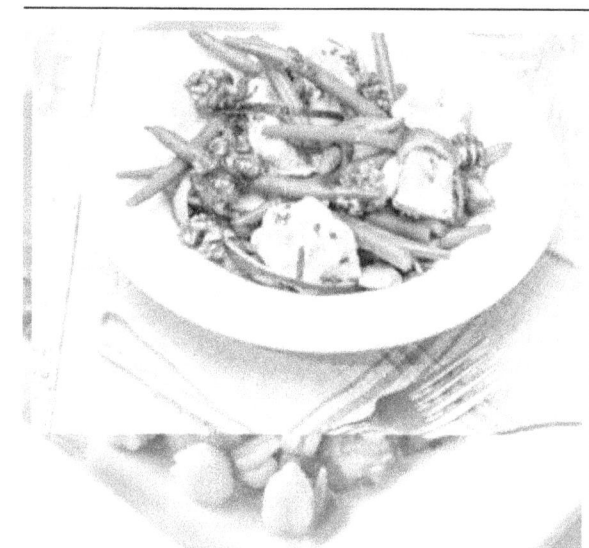

Malta

Malta is a small, flat, limestone-covered island in the Mediterranean Sea. It has a rich history, with traces of Phoenician, Greek, Roman, Byzantine, Arab, and Norman settlements.

Maltese cuisine is a blend of influences from its neighbors, including Italy, Sicily, and North Africa.

Some popular Maltese dishes include pastizzi -savory pastries filled with cheese or peas, rabbit stew, and qaqocc mimli -fish pie. Maltese wines, such as Marsovin and Delicata, are also popular.

It is famous for beaches and its relaxed Mediterranean lifestyle.

INGREDIENTS

- White butter beans 1 cup.
- Green onions 2 chopped.
- Garlic cloves 2 crushed.
- Black olives 10 sliced.
- Fresh parsley 1 cup.
- Dressing
- Apple cider vinegar 1/4 cup.
- Olive oil 1/4 cup.
- Salt and Pepper to taste

DIRECTIONS

- Mix all ingredients and serve chill.

Section V

Fruit Salads

Honduras: Waldorf salad

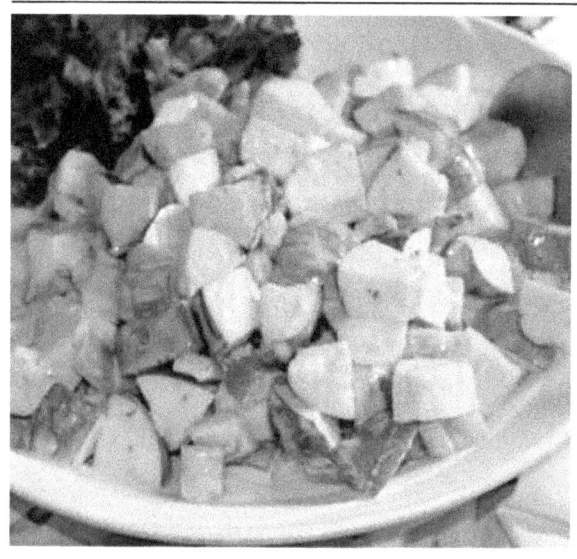

Honduras

Honduras is in Central America. The capital of Honduras is Tegucigalpa.
Honduran cuisine is a blend of indigenous, Spanish, and African influences. Some popular Honduran dishes include baleadas (tortillas filled with beans, cheese, and other toppings), carne asada (grilled meat), and platanos fritos (fried plantains). Honduran beers, such as Salva Vida and Port Royal, are also popular.

INGREDIENTS

- Celery 1/2 cup
- Red grapes 1/2 cup
- Green apples diced
- Mayonnaise 1 cup.
- Sour cream 1/2 cup.
- Salt 1/4 teaspoon
- Crushed black pepper 1/4 teaspoon

DIRECTIONS

- Mix all ingredients. Season with salt and pepper.

Uruguay: Uruguay Salad

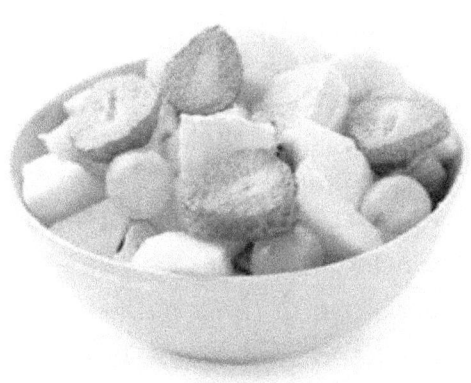

Uruguay

Uruguay is a located in South America. The capital of Uruguay is Montevideo. Popular Uruguayan dishes include asado (grilled meat), chivito (a sandwich made with grilled steak, ham, and cheese), and pastel de papas (a baked dish made with potatoes, onions, and meat). Uruguayan beers, such as Patricia and Pilsen, are also popular.

The country is known for its natural beauty, with a number of national parks and reserves, such as the Lagoons of Rocha and the Punta del Este.

INGREDIENTS

- Pineapple 1 cup
- Melon 1 sliced
- Mango 1 chopped.
- Bananas 2 sliced
- Kiwis 1 sliced
- Lemon juice 2-tab spoon
- Brown sugar tab 2-tab spoon.
- Orange juice 1/2 cup.

DIRECTIONS

- Mix lemon juice, ginger powder, orange juice, and brown sugar in a bowl and set aside.
- Mix all fruits and stir in lemon juice dressing.
- Sprinkle coconut on top.
- Serve immediately.

Venezuela: Venezuela Salad

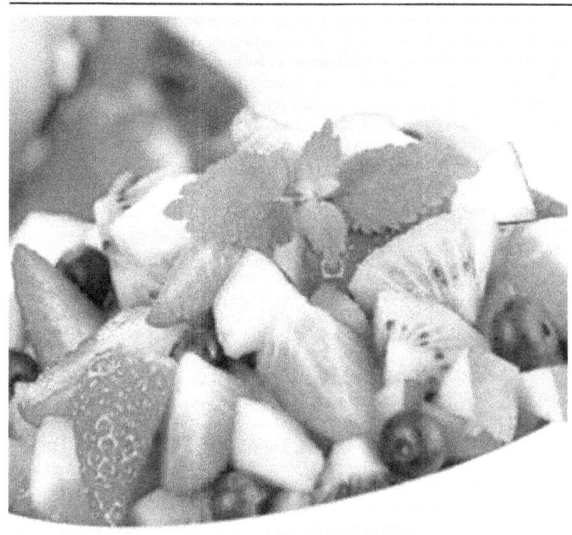

INGREDIENTS

- Blueberries 2 cups sliced.
- Strawberries washed, cut, and sliced 2 cups.
- Banana 2 sliced.
- Asian pear cut into chunks.
- Fresh lime juice 2 tabspoon.
- Honey 2 tabspoon.

Venezuela

Venezuela is a country located in South America. The capital of Venezuela is Caracas. Venezuela has a tropical climate, with hot and humid weather year-round. Popular Venezuelan dishes include arepas (corn cakes filled with various toppings), pabellón criollo (a dish made with rice, black beans, and shredded beef), and hallacas (cornmeal dough filled with meat and vegetables, wrapped in a banana leaf). Venezuelan beers, such as Polar and Regional, are also popular.

Angel Falls (the highest waterfall in the world), Los Roques archipelago, and The Andes Mountains are some famous tourist attractions.

Venezuela is also home to a number of cultural and historical landmarks, such as the National Pantheon, the National Theater, and the Plaza Bolivar.

DIRECTIONS

- Mix honey and lime juice. Salad dressing is ready.
- Mix all fruits, and drizzle salad dressing.
- Chill for 1 hour and then serve

Cayman Islands: Cayman Islands Salad

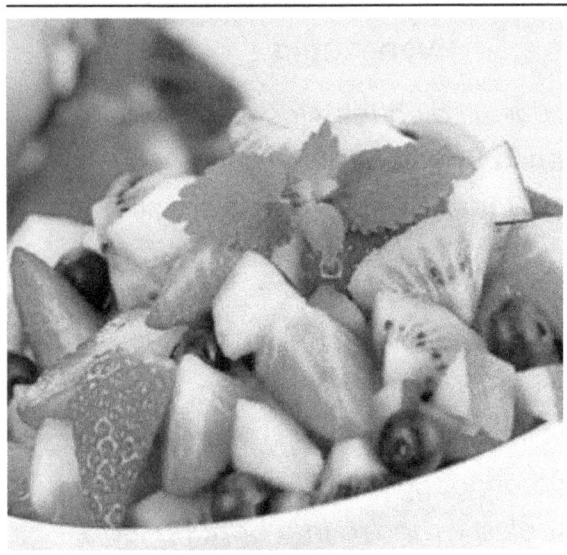

INGREDIENTS

- Avocados 2 peeled and mashed
- Orange juice 1/2 cup
- Grated orange rind 1 tab spoon.
- Honey 3 tab spoon
- Sugar 1 teaspoon.
- Strawberries 3 sliced
- Honeydew melon 1/4 cup
- Watermelon pieces 1/4 cup.
- Oranges sliced 1/2 cups

Cayman Islands

The Cayman Islands, islands in the Caribbean Ocean. The primary fascination in Cayman is the water. Swimming and diving draw numerous guests every year. The capital of the Cayman Islands is George Town.

Popular food and beverages of the Cayman Islands include stew, coconut shrimp, heavy cake, lemonade, watermelon lush, and alcohol.

Coral reefs, underwater sculptures, beautiful beaches and clear waters have made this island a favorite among visitors.

DIRECTIONS

- Mix mashed avocado honey, orange juice, lemon juice, and cream in a bowl and chill.
- Mix strawberries, honeydew melon, oranges, and watermelon slices to the mashed avocado bowl.
- Chill and enjoy!

Saint Kitts And Nevis: Chicken and mixed fruit salad

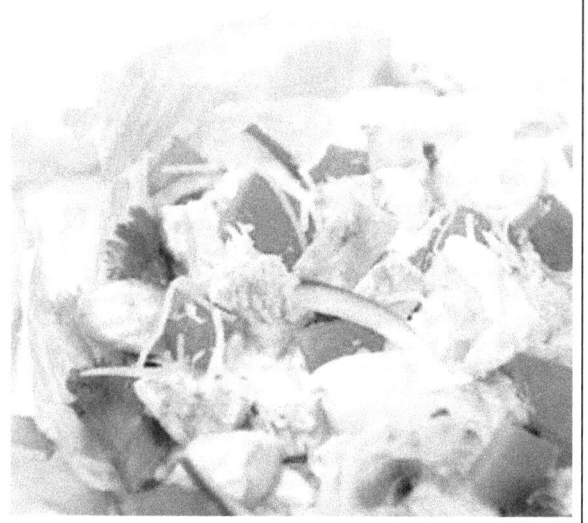

Saint Kitts And Nevis

It is a country located in the Lesser Antilles in the Eastern Caribbean Sea. Its capital is Basseterre

Saint Kitts and Nevis is made up of two main islands, Saint Kitts and Nevis, and a number of small islets

Popular dishes are roti, dark pudding, conch fritters, and Johnny cakes. Ting 'n Sting is tasty drink for a sunny day.

Fun activity include Diving & bird watching are truly remarkable on Saint Kitts and Nevis for tourists.

INGREDIENTS

- Shredded boiled chicken 2 cups
- Shallots 2 finely chopped.
- Celery 2 stalks thinly sliced.
- Crisp lettuce 3 leaves tear into pieces.
- Mandarins 3 peeled and sliced.
- Apple 1
- Pineapple slices 2
- Chives chopped 1 tab spoon.
- Cream 2 tab spoon.
- Tangy mayonnaise 1/2 cup
- Lemon juice 2 tab spoon.
- Salt 1/2 teaspoon.
- Lemon pepper 1/4 teaspoon

DIRECTIONS

- Mix shredded chicken, celery, torn lettuce leaves, Apple slices, salt, shallot, mandarins, pineapple slices, lemon juice, and lemon pepper.
- Add mayonnaise and cream and toss well.
- Garnish with fresh chives and serve

Turks and Caicos Islands: Island Salad

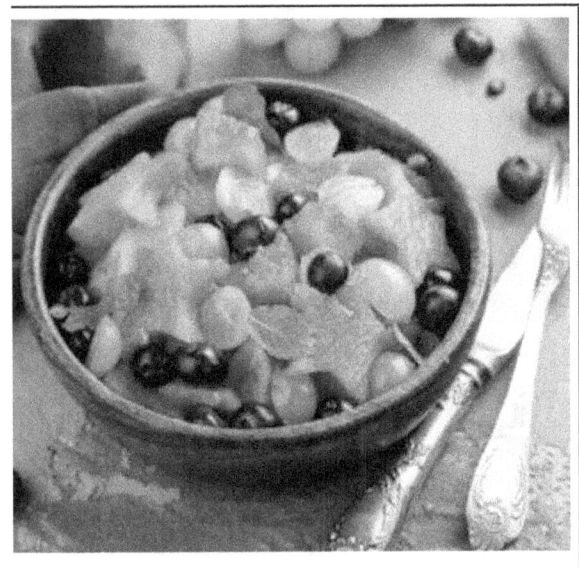

INGREDIENTS

- Mango 2 sliced
- Papaya diced 1 cup
- Kiwi 1 sliced
- Dragon fruit or strawberries diced 1/2 cup
- Watermelon 1 cup cubes
- Pineapple 1 cup cubes
- Banana 2 sliced
- For dressing.
- Honey 2-tab spoon
- Lime zest of 1 lime, about 1 teaspoon.
- Lime juice 2-tab spoon.
- Roasted coconut 2 tabs poon.
- Fresh mint for garnishing.

Turks and Caicos Islands

The archipelago comprises two islands, the Turks islands and the Caicos Islands. Popular Seafood-lobster, crab and rice. Islander Ginger Lager is considered as the best beverage on the island. Activities include scuba diving, swimming, sailing, parasailing, and fishing.

DIRECTIONS

- Mix lime juice, lime zest, and honey in a bowl.
- Mix all fruits. Drizzle dressing and toss well.

Saint Martin: Tropical Fruit Salad

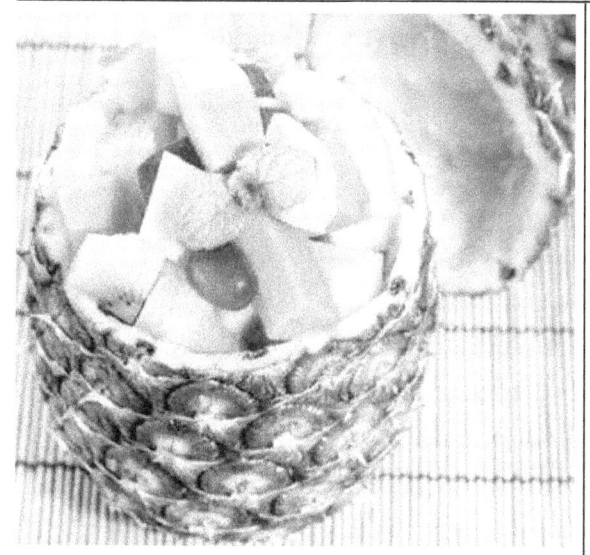

INGREDIENTS

- 12 Mandarin oranges (fresh) 2 cups
- Strawberries sliced 1/4 cup.
- Fresh pineapple cubes 1/2 cup.
- Kiwi sliced 5 halved
- Bananas 2 sliced
- 3 mangos cut in chunks

DRESSING:

- Lemon zest 1 teaspoon.
- Lime juice 2 tab spoon.
- Mandarins juice ¼ cup.
- Honey 1/4 Cup.
- Fresh grated ginger 1/2 teaspoon.
- Poppy seeds 1 teaspoon.

Saint Martin

Saint Martin is an island in the Caribbean that is divided between the French collectivity of Saint-Martin and the Dutch territory of Saint Maarten. Philipsburg is the capital of Saint Martin.

The island is known for its sandy rocks, 37 beaches, fish, and beautiful harbors. Popular roadside food trucks, which mostly include Chicken sate and Soato Soup with un activities including Swimming and Sunbathing.

DIRECTIONS

- Mix all dressing ingredients.
- Combine all fruits, and pour dressing.
- Refrigerate for 1 hour.

British Virgin Islands: BVI Salad

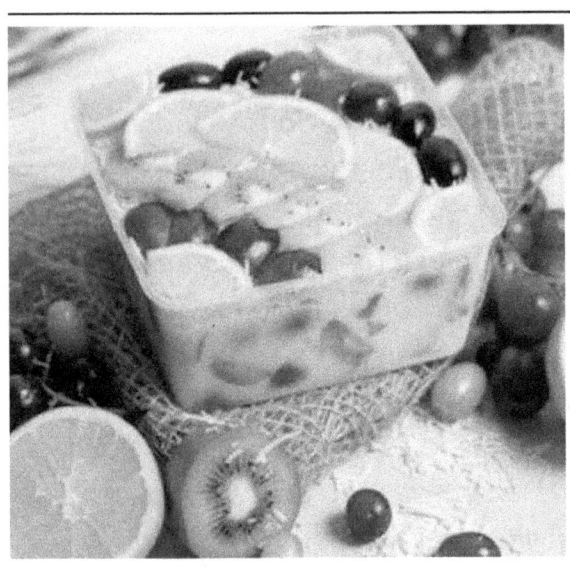

British Virgin Islands

Road Town is the capital of BVI. Popular dishes include Fish chowder, snapper, whelks, mussel pie, conch stew and shark is a few of the most loved food varieties of these islands.
Rum, mixed drinks, and cocktails are the most popular drinks of this island.
Enjoy the natural beauty, and a friendly atmosphere, of this island.

INGREDIENTS

- Bananas, sliced 2
- Kiwi fruit cubes 2
- Medium mango, peeled and cubed 1
- Pina colada yogurt 1/2 cup
- Pineapple slices ½ cup.
- Sweetened shredded coconut, toasted 1/2 cup.

DIRECTIONS

- Mix all fruits and pinacolada yogurt.
- Sprinkle coconut and serve

Anguilla: Anguilla Salad

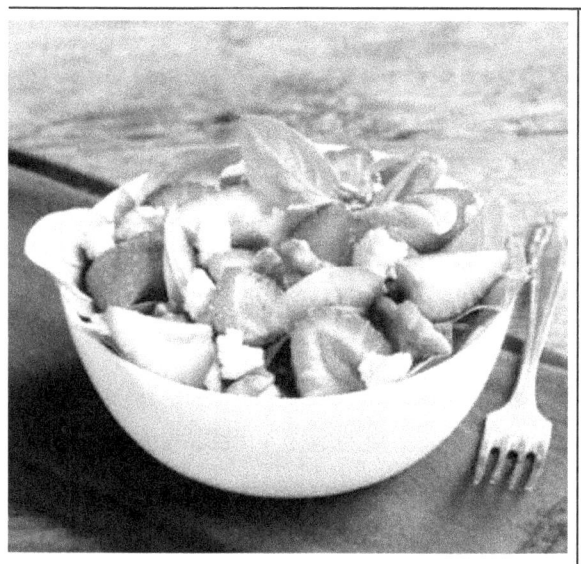

INGREDIENTS

- Frozen unsweetened strawberries 2 cups
- Bananas 2 sliced
- Fresh blueberries 1/2 cup
- Peach pie filling 1 can
- Green grapes ½ cup
- 3/4 cup green grapes
- 1 can (21 ounces) peach pie filling

Anguilla

Anguilla is a ravishing little island in the Eastern Caribbean Sea and is a British Overseas Territory. The capital of Anguilla is The Valley.

The Rum Punch cocktail and Pigeon peas and rice are often considered as the signature food and drink of the island.

This is a place with gorgeous bays, some of the best white-sanded beaches in the world, palm trees and the turquoise ocean all around. Some famous tourist attraction points are Rendezvous Bay, Little Bay, Crocus Bay, Shoal Bay, Savanna Bay, Scrub and Sandy islands. In short, Anguilla is a fine destination for scuba diving or snorkeling.

DIRECTIONS

- Mix all fruits and refrigerate for 1 hour
- Enjoy!

Syria: Syrian Salad

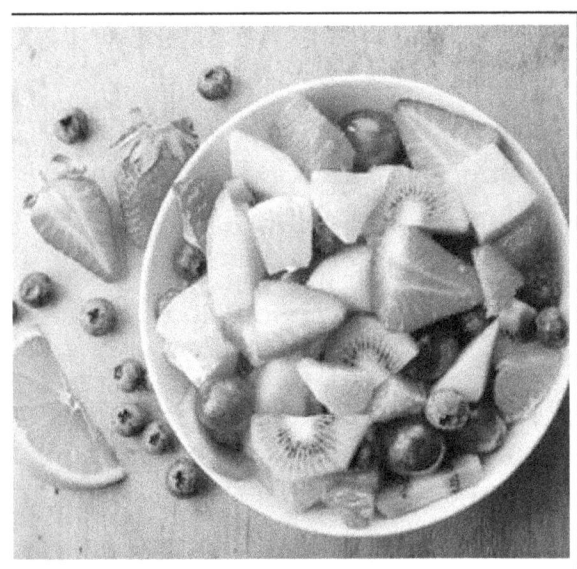

INGREDIENTS

- Dried apricot 1/4 cup.
- Dried figs 1/4 cup
- Prunes 1/4 cup.
- Raisins 1/4 cup.
- Chopped walnuts 1 cup
- Chopped almonds 1 cup
- Pine nuts 1 cup.
- Sugar 2 tab spoon
- Rosewater 2 tab spoon.

Syria

Syria is located in the Middle East. Syria has a rich cultural heritage and history.
The capital of Syria is Damascus. It is one of the oldest continuously inhabited cities in the world.
The most famous dishes and drinks is the Kebab, Hummus and Baba Ghanoush dip sauces, Syrian coffee, and Arak.

DIRECTIONS

- Leave dried fruits in water for 48 hours.
- Mix remaining ingredients and chill

Yemen: Yemen Salad

Yemen

Yemen is located in Middle East, on the southwestern tip of the Arabian Peninsula. The capital of Yemen is Sana'a. It is the largest city in the country.

Yemen is also known for its aromatic and flavorful spices.

Famous spices from Yemen include cardamom, cumin, and coriander.

Yemeni coffee is traditionally grown in the highlands of the country and is considered to be some of the best in the world.

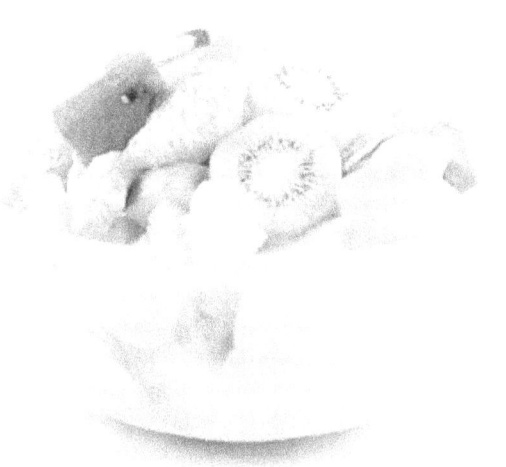

INGREDIENTS

- Milk 1 cup
- Yogurt 1/2 cup
- Bell pepper
- Cumin 1/2 teaspoon.
- Green chili 1
- Garlic 1 clove
- Mint leaves 1/4 cup.
- Lime juice 2 tabspoon.
- Arabic flat bread

DIRECTIONS

- Blend bell pepper, garlic, chili, lime juice, cumin, salt, and mint, whisk milk and yogurt and add blended mint mixture.
- Place flatbread pieces on a serving dish.
- Pour milk mixture and let it rest for 5 minutes.
- Garnish with pomegranate seeds
- Chill and enjoy!

Asia

South Korea: South Korea Salad

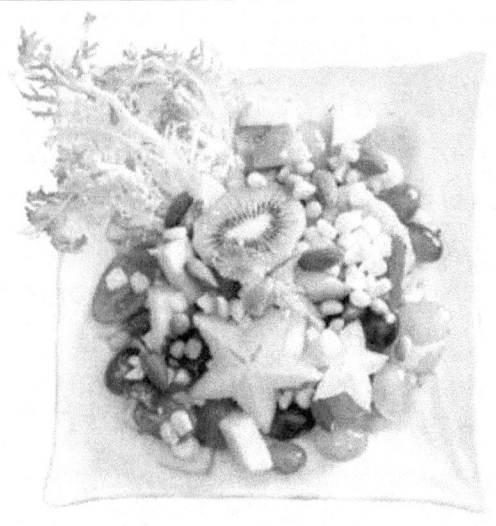

INGREDIENTS

- Grapes
- Korean Pear 1 sliced
- Apple 1 sliced
- Hard-boiled eggs 3
- Roasted peanuts or almonds ¼ cup
- Lemon juice 2 tabspoon
- Salt 1/4 teaspoon
- Black pepper 1/4 teaspoon.

South Korea

South Korea, is in East Asia, the capital city of South Korea is Seoul.

Korean barbecue, kimchi, bibimbap, green tea, coffee, and yakult are some favourite dishes and beverages of South Korea.

South Korea is a has a diverse landscape, ranging from rugged mountains to coastal areas.

It is home to a number of natural parks and protected areas, including the Seoraksan National Park, which is known for its beautiful mountain scenery.

DIRECTIONS

- Mix all fruits.
- Add lemon juice, salt, black pepper and mix well
- Serve chilled.

Asia

Brunei: Brunei Salad

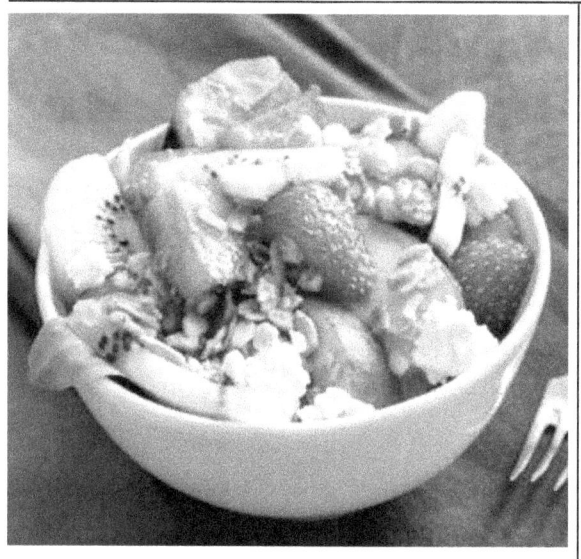

INGREDIENTS

For the fruit salad
- Pineapple 1 cube
- Cucumber 1 sliced
- Green pear 1 sliced
- Apple 1sliced
- Papaya cubed, 1 cup

For the Peanut Sauce
- Water ½ cup
- Tamarind paste 1 tab spoon.
- Peanut butter 2 tab spoon
- Crushed red chili 1 tab spoon.
- Brown sugar 1/4 cup.
- Banana 1 sliced.

Brunei

Brunei is a small, oil-rich country located on the island of Borneo in Southeast Asia. The capital city of Brunei is Bandar Seri Begawan.

Laksa (spicy noodle soup), Nasi katok (dish of rice with meat), Satay (skewered meat), Sireh (traditional drink made from the sap of the sireh plant) are some famous foods and drinks influenced by the indigenous Malay culture.

Beautiful attractions include beaches, rainforests, and the Royal Regalia Museum.

DIRECTIONS

- Blend sauce ingredients in a blender.
- Mix all fruits.
- Pour peanut sauce dressing on salad fruits and toss well.

Solomon Islands: Solomon Islands Salad

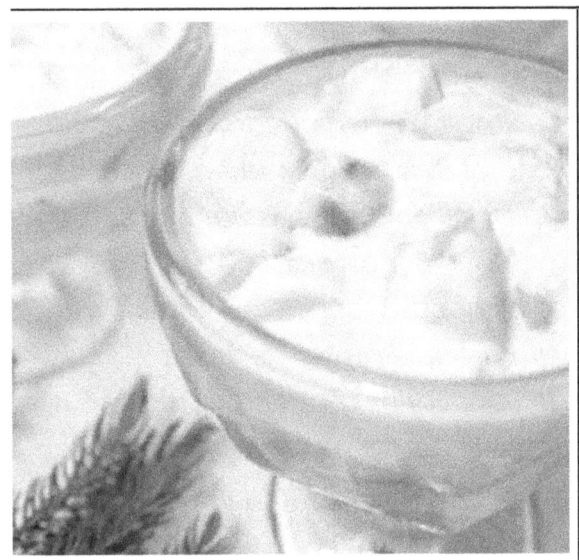

INGREDIENTS

- Mangoes 2 chopped
- Bananas 3 sliced
- Cherry chopped ¼ cup
- Pineapple chopped 1/2 cup.
- Peaches 2 chopped
- purple grapes 1/4
- cup sliced
- Kiwi fruit 1 sliced.
- Fresh basil leaves ½ cup.
- Greek yogurt 1 cup
- Roasted Chopped pistachios ½ cup.
- Basil sugar
- Fresh basil leaves 3
- Sugar 2-tab spoon

Solomon Islands

The Solomon Islands, located in the southern Pacific Ocean, consists of five main islands: Guadalcanal, Honiara, Malaita, Santa Isabel, and San Cristobal
and over 900 smaller islands in Oceania
The capital is Honiara.
It has a diverse culture and cuisine, influenced by the Melanesian, Polynesian, and Asian heritage, which includes sago, taro, and grilled chicken.
Tea, beer, and kava are famous refreshing drinks of the Solomon Islands.
The Solomon Islands are known for their beautiful beaches, crystal clear waters, and rich cultural and historical heritage.

DIRECTIONS

- Blend basil leaves and granulated sugar
- Combine all fruits.
- Sprinkle basil sugar.
- Add yogurt and mix well all ingredients.
- Chill for 1 hour and then serve.

Tonga: Tonga Salad

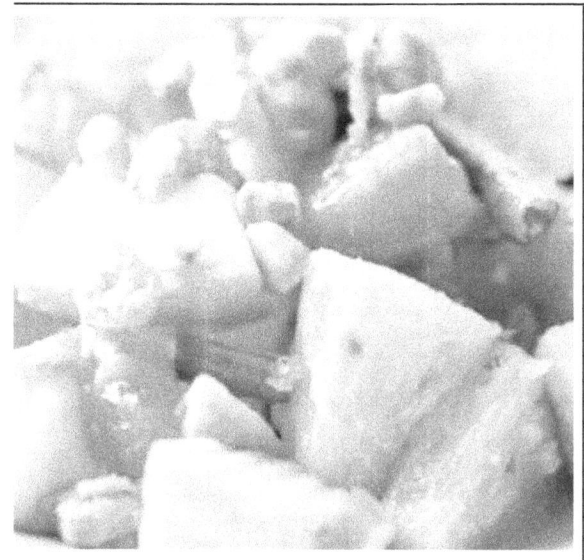

INGREDIENTS

- Mango 1 chopped
- Bananas 3 sliced
- Pineapple 2 cups
- Lemon juice 3-tab spoon
- Shredded coconut 4-tab spoon.

Tonga

Tonga is a country situated in the southwestern Pacific Ocean. It comprises of 170 islands divided into three islands. Groups. Ha'apai in the centre, Tongatapu in the south, and Vava'u in the north.
Popular food and drinks of these islands include fish, taro, sago, tea, and kava. Fresh fruits, includes mangoes, papayas, pineapples, and coconuts.
Tonga is known for its beautiful beaches, clear waters, and rich cultural and historical heritage.

DIRECTIONS

- Mix fruits, coconut, and lime juice
- Chill for 2 hours and then serve

Vanuatu: Vanuatu Salad

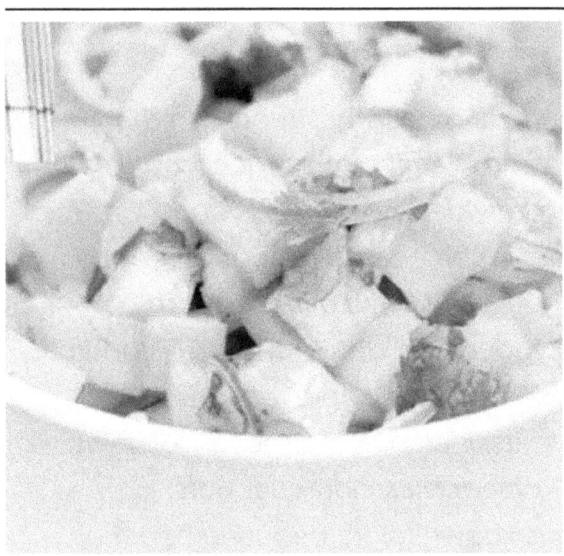

INGREDIENTS

- Green papaya 1 cup.
- Chopped peanuts 1 cup
- Frozen shredded coconut 1 cup
- Green onion 1 chopped.
- Vegetable oil 2 tab spoon.
- Lime juice 2 tab spoon.
- Salt ¼ teaspoon.
- Black pepper ¼ teaspoon

Vanuatu

Vanuatu is a Polynesian island country located in the South Pacific Ocean. Some traditional dishes include coconut crab, fish, and wild boar.

Some popular drinks in Vanuatu are kava, coconut water, fruit juices, and locally brewed beer.

Vanuatu is known for its tropical climate, beautiful beaches, and rich history. Tourists enjoy swimming, hiking and nature walks in Vanuatu. The country is also an important center for ecotourism, as it is home to many unique plant and animal species.

DIRECTIONS

- Mix all ingredients, and sprinkle salt and pepper.
- Black pepper ¼ teaspoon

South Sudan: South Sudan Salad

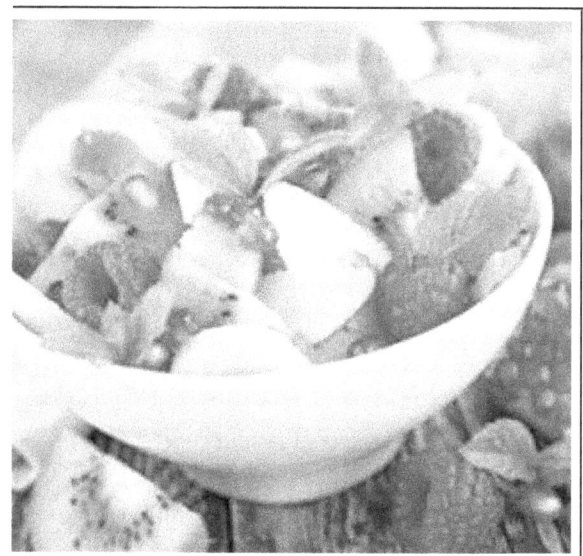

INGREDIENTS

- Avocado 1 peeled and sliced
- Peach 1 sliced
- Guava 1 sliced
- Banana 2
- Papaya 1 cup
- Pear 1
- Mango 1
- Pineapple.1/2 cup
- Lemon juice 1/4 cup
- Freshly grated coconut as per need
- Roasted peanuts chopped as per need
- Honey 1 teaspoon

South Sudan

South Sudan is located in the East African region.

South Sudan is a country located in East Africa. It is the largest country in Africa by land area and is home to a population of around 12 million people. Juba is the largest and capital city of this country.

Some traditional foods in South Sudan are peanut butter, roasted and grilled meat, esh (a kind of porridge).

Drinks in South Sudan include tea, coffee, and a variety of fruit juices. Alcoholic beverages, including beer and traditional brews made from sorghum or millet, are also popular.

South Sudan is home to a variety of wildlife, including elephants, lions, giraffes, and a wide range of bird species and is also home to the Nile River, the longest river in Africa and a major water source for the region.

DIRECTIONS

- Mix all fruits in a serving bowl.
- Add lemon juice.
- Garnish with coconut and roasted peanuts

Sudan: Canned fruit salad

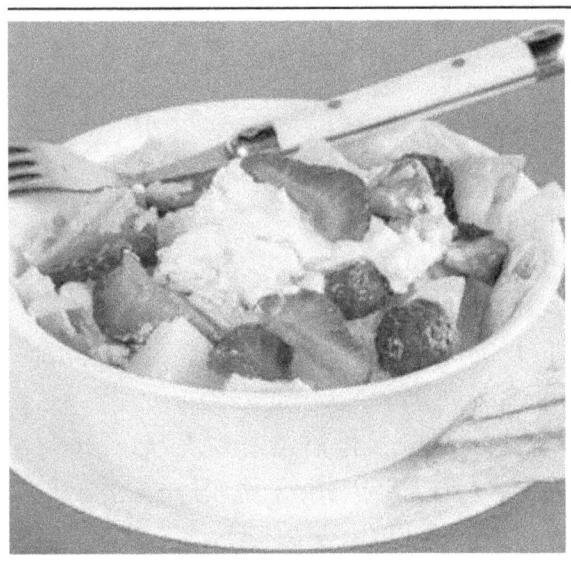

Sudan

Sudan is a country located in Northeast Africa. Sudan has a rich history and was once home to ancient civilizations such as the Kingdom of Kush.
The capital is Khartoum.
Famous food and drinks include Bazeen (porridge), Karkad (drink made from hibiscus flowers), Dukhun (spice blend made with cumin, coriander, and other spices)

INGREDIENTS

- Canned pineapple cubes 2 cups
- Orange 1
- Mango 1
- Banana 2
- Lemon juice 2 tab spoon
- Brown sugar 1 tab spoon
- Roasted coconut 1 cup.

DIRECTIONS

- Mix all fruits. Add lemon juice and roasted coconut, and mix.

Cape Verde: Cape Verde Salad

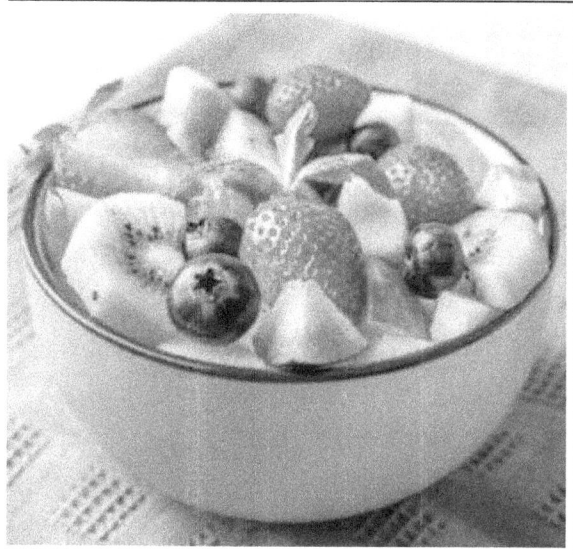

Cape Verde

Cabo Verde (also known as Cape Verde) is a country located in West Africa, made up of a group of islands in the Atlantic Ocean. Known for its beautiful beaches, vibrant culture, and rich history.
Popular dishes and drinks include grilled seafood, tuna, swordfish, and shrimp and rinks- ginger beer, cashew wine, and grogue. Lots of fresh fruits, such as mangoes, papayas, and bananas.

INGREDIENTS

- Kiwi fruit 2 peeled and sliced 2
- Passion fruit pulp 2 cups
- Pineapple puree 1 cup.
- Papaya small cubes
- Mango ripe 2
- Water 1 cup
- Honey 1/4 cup.
- Lemon juice 1 tab spoon
- Lime juice 1 tab spoon.

DIRECTIONS

- Add passion fruit pulp, pineapple slices, water, honey, lime juice, and lemon juice in a blender and blend well.
- Fruit dressing is ready.
- Mix remaining fruits, add fruit dressing, and toss well
- Serve chill.

Libya: Libya Salad

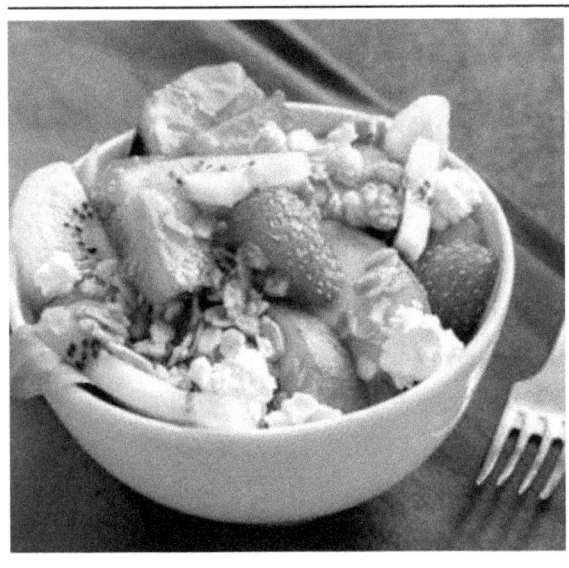

INGREDIENTS

- Dried fruits like apricot and figs 1 cup
- Chopped blanched almonds or pine nuts ¼ cup.
- Banana 1
- Chopped raisins s 1 cup.
- Orange blossom water 2 tab spoon.
- Crushed coconut for garnishing.

Libya

Libya is located in North Africa. It is known for its rich history and cultural heritage.
Libya is home to a large portion of the Sahara desert, which is the largest desert in the world.
Tripoli is the capital of Libya. It has a rich cultural heritage influenced by African, Arab, and Mediterranean traditions.
Popular dishes are shawarma and kebabs.
Tea is prefer drink
The Libyan coast is home to a number of beautiful beaches and resorts, which are popular with tourists.

DIRECTIONS

- Add raisins, chopped figs, apricot in a bowl. Add 2 cups of water and bring it to a boil for 10 minutes on low flame.
- Then cool this mixture at room temperature and chill for 1 hour.
- Add banana slices, orange blossom water, pine nuts and mix well.
- Sprinkle with desiccated coconut.

Nunavut Canada: Chicken and mixed fruit salad

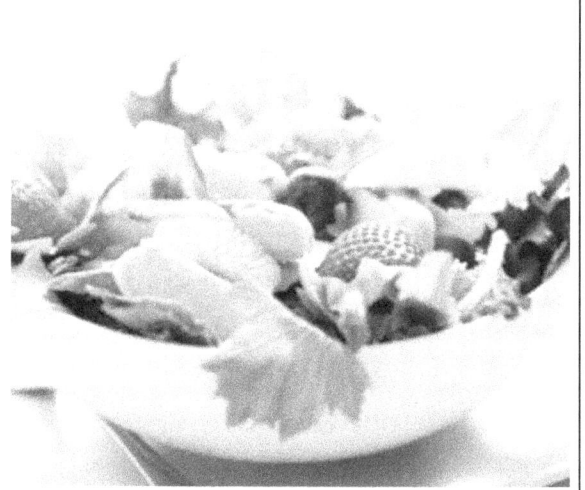

INGREDIENTS

- Shredded boiled chicken 2 cups
- Shallots 2 finely chopped.
- Celery 2 stalks thinly sliced.
- Crisp lettuce 3 leaves tear into pieces.
- Mandarins 3 peeled and sliced.
- Apple 1
- Pineapple slices 2
- Chives chopped 1 tab spoon.
- Cream 2 tab spoon.
- Tangy mayonnaise 1/2 cup
- Lemon juice 2 tab spoon.
- Salt 1/2 teaspoon.
- Lemon pepper 1/4 teaspoon

Nunavut, Canada

The largest and most northern territory in Canada, Nunavut.
The capital of Nunavut is Iqaluit.
Traditional Inuit food in Nunavut includes a variety of meats such as caribou, seal, and Arctic char.
Qaggiq and labmajuq are considered as traditional drinks of Nunavut.
Nunavut is located in the Arctic region of Canada, and it is known for its rugged, remote landscape, which includes tundra, mountains, and glaciers. The territory is home to a number of wildlife species, including polar bears, caribou, and arctic foxes.

DIRECTIONS

- Mix shredded chicken, celery, tear lettuce leaves, Apple slices, salt, shallot, mandarins, pineapple slices, lemon juice, and lemon pepper.
- Add mayonnaise, cream, and toss well.
- Garnish with fresh chives and serve

Puebla, Mexico: Cinnamon apple salad

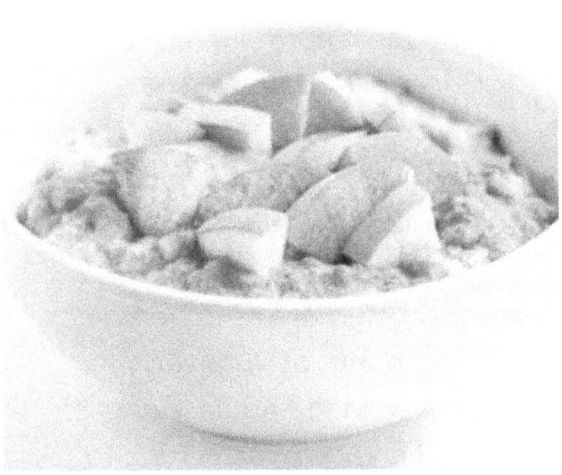

Puebla, Mexico

Puebla, in central Mexico that is known for its rich history, food, culture, and tradition. The capital is Puebla, and it is located in the southeast of Mexico City.

Puebla is known for its rich culinary traditions, popular Mexican dishes and drinks are mole poblano and chiles en nogada, coffee, tea, soda, beer,

tequila and mezcal,

Its beautiful landscapes, which include mountains, forests, and beaches.

Puebla is home to a number historical sites; Great Pyramid of Cholula, which is the largest pyramid in the world by volume.

INGREDIENTS

- Apples 3 sliced
- Lemon juice 1-tab spoon
- Butter 2-tab spoon.
- Sugar 1-tab spoon
- White wine 1/4 cup.
- Cinnamon 1 teaspoon
- Chopped walnuts or almonds
- Whipped cream 1/2 cup

DIRECTIONS

- Melt butter in a pan.
- Add apples, lemon juice and simmer for 1 minute.
- Mix cinnamon, vinegar, cover and simmer for 5 minutes or until Apple gets soft.
- Garnish with chopped nuts and whipped cream.

Playa del Carmen, Mexico: Special avocado salad

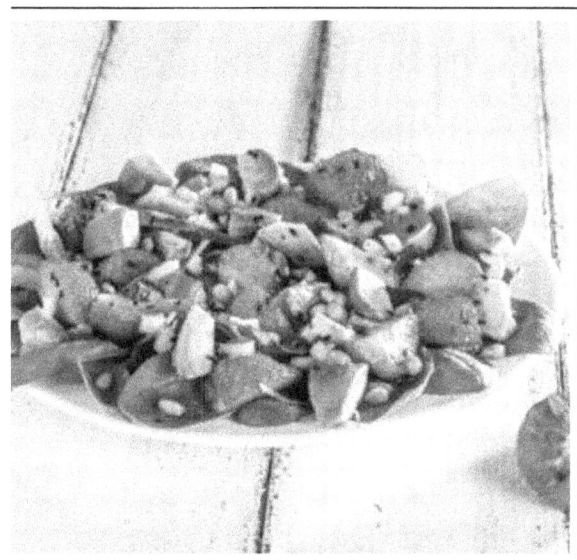

INGREDIENTS

- Avocados 2 peeled and mashed
- Orange juice 1 /2 cup
- Grated orange rind 1 tabspoon.
- Honey 3 tabspoon
- Sugar 1 teaspoon.
- Strawberries 3 sliced
- Honey dew melon 1/4 cup
- Water melon pieces 1/4 cup.
- Oranges sliced 1/2 cup

Playa del Carmen, Mexico

The city, Playa del Carmen, is a popular tourist destination known for its beautiful beaches, crystal-clear waters, and tropical climate.

Playa del Carmen is located on the Caribbean coast of the Yucatán Peninsula in Mexico.

Tacos, Enchiladas, and tamales are some famous cuisines of this city.

Some of the most popular drinks in Playa del Carmen include margaritas, cocktails made with tequila or mezcal, and Mexican beers such as Corona and Tecate.

Playa del Carmen is also home to a number of cultural and historical attractions, including the ancient Maya ruins of Tulum and the Xcaret eco-archeological park.

DIRECTIONS

- Mix mashed avocado honey,orange juice ,lemon juice and cream in a bowl and chill.
- Mix strawberries,honey dew melon, oranges, watermelon slices to the mashed avocado bowl.
- Chill and enjoy!

Philadelphia, PA: Cream cheese fruit salad

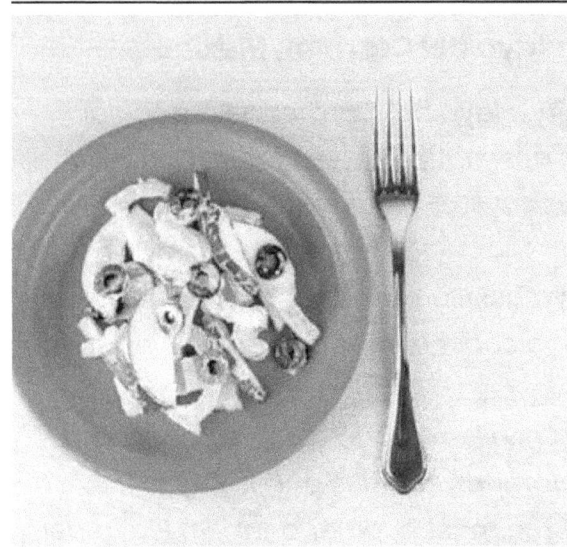

Philadelphia, PA

Philadelphia, Pennsylvania, is a city located in the southeastern United States. Philadelphia has been called "The birthplace of America"

Philadelphia is also known for its diverse cuisine, which includes a range of traditional and modern dishes, which include Cheesesteak, Hoagie sandwich, and Soft pretzel.

Philadelphia is home to the Philadelphia Stock Exchange, the world's oldest stock exchange.

INGREDIENTS

- Strawberries sliced ½ cup.
- Apple diced 2
- Pineapple chopped ½ cup
- Peaches diced 2
- Cream cheese ½ cup
- Mayonnaise ¼ cup
- Cream ¼ cup
- Lemon juice 2 tabspoon.
- Chopped nuts 4 tabspoon

DIRECTIONS

- Add all fruits in a bowl.
- Stir in mayonnaise, cream and cream cheese
- Mix and chill for 1 hour
- Sprinkle chopped nuts before serving.

France: French fruit salad

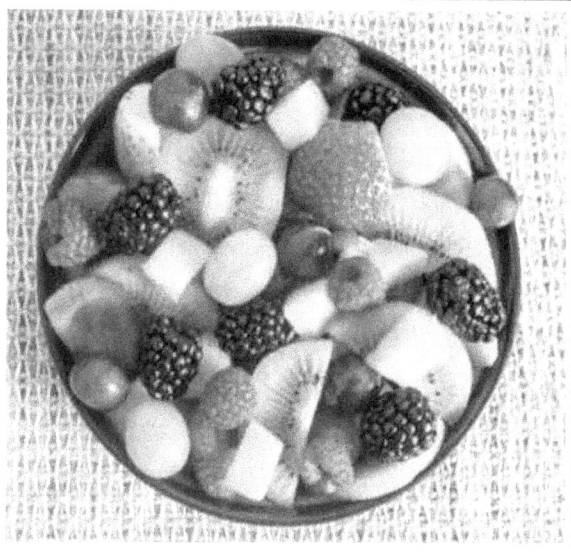

INGREDIENTS

- 1 banana
- 1 orange
- Grape fruit 1 cup
- Pineapple slices 1 cup.
- Lemon juice 2 tabspoon.
- Candied raisins and fruits.
- Seasonal fruits I use peaches, plums and apricot.
- Rum 1 cup.

France

France is in Western Europe, its capital in Paris.

France is also famous for its cuisine and wine, dishes such as escargot, coq au vin, and croissants.

French wine is known for its variety and quality; it is home to many famous landmarks and museums.

The Mona Lisa and The Eiffel Tower are famous symbols of this country.

French fashion is known for its famous fashion designers. Sophistication and style, and many

DIRECTIONS

- Mix all fruits.
- Add lemon juice and toss well.
- Refrigerate for 1 hour.

Belarus: Belarus Fresh Strawberries

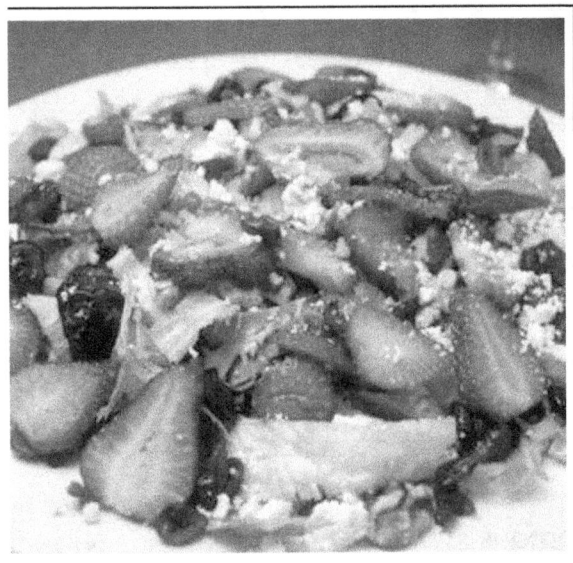

INGREDIENTS

- Sviežaja klubnicy
- Strawberries washed and sliced 2 cups
- Sugar 1 teaspoon.

Belarus

Belarus is in Eastern Europe. The capital of Belarus is Minsk. Traditional Belarusian dishes often feature potatoes, beetroots, and other vegetables, as well as meat and dairy products. Popular Belarusian foods and drinks are Draniki, Kvas, Vatrushka, and Borscht. Belarus has a diverse landscape, with forests, marshes, and rolling hills. The country is known for its many lakes and rivers, and it has a number of protected areas and national parks. The Belavezhskaya Pushcha National Park, which is home to a number of rare and endangered species.

DIRECTIONS

- Add strawberries in a bowl, sprinkle some sugar and mix gently.
- Enjoy this super easy and delicious strawberry salad.

Europe

Kosovo: Kosovo Salad

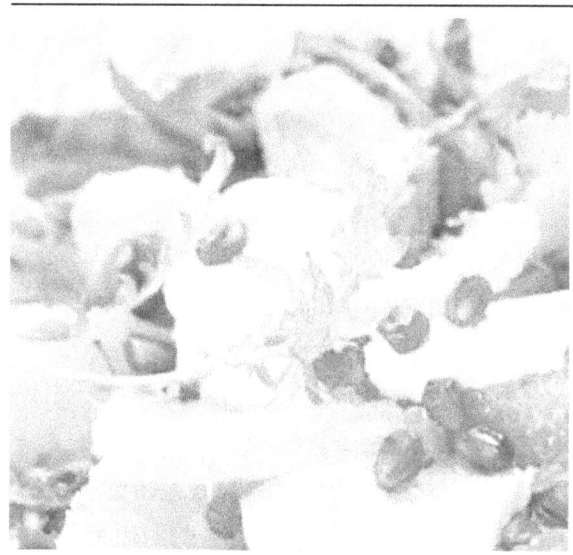

Kosovo

*Kosovo is a.
Kosovo is in the Western Balkans region of Europe. The capital of Kosovo is Pristina. It is known for its production of textiles, minerals, and energy.
Cevapi (a type of grilled sausage), Tavë Kosi (rice and meat dish), Burek (a savory pastry), and Rakija (a type of brandy) are some famous foods and beverages of Kosovo.
Kosovo has a diverse landscape, with mountains, forests, and valleys and has a rich cultural heritage of music, dance, and folk traditions.*

INGREDIENTS

- Oranges sliced 2 peeled and sliced into thin discs
- Feta cheese crumbled 1/2 cup.
- Black olives 10.
- Hard boiled eggs 3
- Lemon peeled and sliced 1
- Fresh mint leaves.
- Olive oil 2 tabspoon.
- Salt 1/4 teaspoon.
- Crushed black pepper 1/4 teaspoon.

DIRECTIONS

- Arrange the slices of lemon,cheese herd boiled eggs slices on a serving platter.
- Add chopped mint
- Top with olives
- Drizzle some olive oil.

Iceland: Fresh Fruit Salad

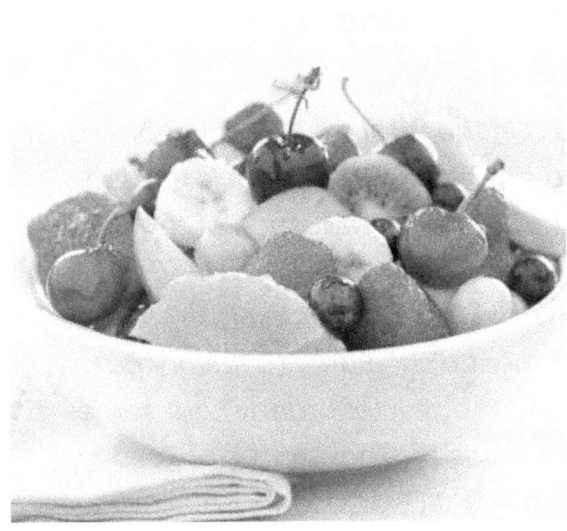

INGREDIENTS

- 1 red or green apple
- 2 tangerines or small oranges, peeled
- 12 black or green grapes
- 1 medium banana, peeled
- 2 kiwi fruits, peeled
- 1 large thick slice of pineapple, fresh or canned
- 1 glass of fresh unsweetened orange juice – you can also use grape, pineapple or apple juice

Iceland

A country located in the North Atlantic Ocean, Iceland. The capital of Iceland is Reykjavik.

Fish, Rye bread, skyr, and hot dogs are famous cuisines of Iceland. Brennivín is a traditional drink and its milk is served as a beverage and is known for its high quality and natural taste.

Iceland has a rich cultural heritage, and it is known for its literature, music, and art. Iceland has a unique and varied landscape, with volcanoes, geysers, hot springs, waterfalls, and glaciers.

It is a country with a strong cultural identity and a rich history, and it is known for its natural beauty and outdoor activities, such as hiking, skiing, and fishing.

DIRECTIONS

- Wash the apple and then cut into quarters removing the core. Cut into chunks
- Divide the tangerines or oranges into segments
- Wash grapes and half each one
- Cut banana and kiwi fruit into slices
- Cut pineapple into chunks
- Place all fruit in the bowl, add the orange juice and mix well

Bulgaria: Bulgaria Papayas Salad

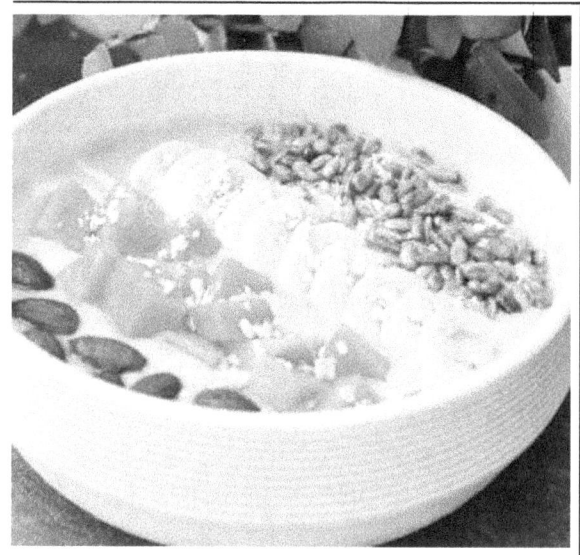

INGREDIENTS

- Baby papayas 2
- Peel, cut and remove seeds.
- Lime 2 sliced.
- Bulgarian yogurt 1 cup.
- Roasted chopped pistachios 1/2 cup.

Bulgaria

Bulgaria is in Southeastern Europe. The capital of Bulgaria is Sofia.

Banitsa (a traditional Bulgarian pastry), Kavarma (a traditional Bulgarian stew), and Tarator (a cold soup) are some famous cuisines of Bulgaria. Bulgaria is also known for its wines, rakia (a type of brandy), and other alcoholic drinks.

Bulgaria has a diverse landscape, with mountains, forests, and beaches, and it is known for its beautiful countryside and charming villages. The country is also home to a number of important cultural and historical sites, such as the Rila Monastery and the Thracian tombs.

DIRECTIONS

- Mix all fruits and yogurt.
- Serve chill.

NEXT STEP

Thanks for purchasing this book, reading it, and taking obedient action as you reflect on your food experiences & relationships. I hope it was enlightening and encouraging and that your life flourishes, one small step and one week at a time.

As you connect with more people & your lifestyle becomes healthier, you will influence many others around you, just like my friends in college influenced me with unique food experiences that led me to create this book.

I would love to hear from you about how this book has impacted you. Your feedback will help me in improving this book and other books in the future.

Receiving your review is important to me, it will help this book reach more people and change lives around the world.

www.ingramcontent.com/pod-product-compliance
Lightning Source LLC
Chambersburg PA
CBHW080458240426
43673CB00005B/230